GANGRENE – CURRENT CONCEPTS AND MANAGEMENT OPTIONS

Edited by **Alexander A. Vitin**

Gangrene – Current Concepts and Management Options
Edited by Alexander A. Vitin

Published by InTech
Janeza Trdine 9, 51000 Rijeka, Croatia

Publishing Process Manager Viktorija Zgela

Technical Editor Teodora Smiljanic

Cover Designer InTech Design Team

Additional hard copies can be obtained from orders@intechopen.com

Gangrene – Current Concepts and Management Options, Edited by Alexander A. Vitin
p. cm.
ISBN 978-953-307-386-6

For EU product safety concerns:
IN TECH d.o.o., Prolaz Marije Krucifikse Kozulić 3, 51000 Rijeka, Croatia,
info@intechopen.com or visit our website at intechopen.com.

Meet the editor

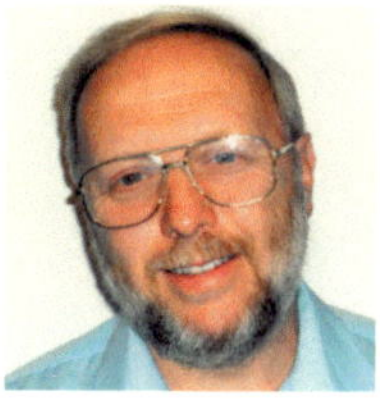

Dr. Alexander A. Vitin, MD, Ph.D. was born on March 03, 1958, in Kharkov, Ukraine. He earned his MD degree from Kharkov High Medical School, University of Kharkov, Ukraine in 1981 and a Ph.D. Degree from the same University in 1985. He worked as a Senior Scientist – Physician at the Central Research Laboratories of the University of Kharkov only to become a Critical Care Fellow in 1986 and then the Attending Physician in the Critical Care Department, Kharkov University Hospital & Trauma Center. From 1990 to 2003 he was an anesthesia resident and the Attending Anesthesiologist and faculty at the Department of Anesthesiology, affiliated with Sackler High Medical School, University of Tel-Aviv, Israel. Since 2003 he holds a position of an Attending Anesthesiologist, Assistant Professor, Division of Transplant Anesthesia, Department of Anesthesiology & Pain Medicine, University of Washington, Seattle, WA, USA.

Contents

Preface

Medicine is the only profession that labours incessantly
to destroy the reason for its own existence.

~James Bryce, 1914

Success of public health programs and advances in modern medicine have substantially increased longevity and survival of sick patients, suffering from various maladies with increased potential of major complications, such as limb and various tissues gangrene.

Gangrene is the term used to describe the necrosis or death of soft tissue due to obstructed circulation, usually followed by decomposition and putrefaction, a serious, potentially fatal complication, that has been well known to generations of physicians for epochs. Despite the immense experience in this field, gained by medicine during its centuries-long history, and impressive recent advances, management of gangrene still presents a significant clinical problem, which is still far from being completely resolved. With ever-growing body of evidence in favor of various treatment modalities, no consensus has been reached so far in respect to superior efficiency of any of the suggested methods. Indeed, even today, with the enormous contemporary armamentarium of treatment methods and immediate access to information literally at his fingertips, a physician, while treating various conditions leading to gangrene/necrosis development, oftentimes faces more unanswered questions than enjoys luxury of choice from plenty of ready-to-use solutions with well-proved efficacy.

In the presented book, the attempt has been made to explore the most important aspects of such detrimental conditions, as are gangrene and necrosis. These included etiology, predisposing factors, demography, pathologic anatomy and mechanisms of development, molecular biology, immunology, microbiology and more. A variety of management strategies, including pharmacological treatment options, surgical and non-surgical solutions and auxiliary methods, are also extensively discussed in the book's chapters. The main goal of this book is not only to provide an easy access to the up-to-date information on the selected topics, but also to help reader to obtain a clear, objective, bias-free and comprehensive picture of the problem.

The presented book lays no claim of encompassing the whole of the problem in all its complexity. Such endeavor would likely have required a multi-volume manuscript.

Rather, the book offers a collection of carefully selected reports of original studies, case presentations and comprehensive review articles, contributed by physicians, who have conducted an extended research in the selected area, experts, who possess a vast, sometimes exquisite experience in practical management of gangrene and necrosis of different locations. The fact that contributors present a variety of clinical disciplines and work in different countries certainly multiplies values of their shared opinions and unique experience.

The presented book contains no unanimously approved recipes and offers no guidelines for immediate implementation. More importantly, the book provides an arena for expert opinions exchange and experience sharing, the approach we believe to be mostly productive, and which we have been following through, while trying to accomplish a task of this book composing and editing.

First part of the book discusses Fournier's gangrene, by far most lethal condition within a spectrum of all maladies complicated by gangrene-necrosis development. This part contains five chapters, discussing in details pathogenesis, diagnosis and natural course of FG, and also treatment options, prognosis and outcome.

Second part, that includes three chapters, is dedicated to the management of intestinal ischemia and bowel necrosis, still difficult-to-diagnose and treat conditions with very high mortality.

Third part contains three chapters, discussing different aspects of diabetic foot gangrene, lung necrosis and also human immunodeficiency-related gangrene.

Fourth part includes two chapters, discussing various aspects of gangrene management, such as antibiotic treatment and hyperbaric oxygen therapy.

I would like to extend my special thanks to all contributors for their outstanding work in putting together a group of such compelling articles, and also for responding to entreaties for revisions and updates with admirable patience and promptness. In particular, I would like to express my deepest appreciation and personal gratitude to Ms. Viktorija Zgela, without whose devotion, tireless, incessantly intense work, continuous help, support and valuable advise this book, most certainly, would never make its way to readers.

We hope that this book will help readers in expanding their knowledge and provide some new ideas for further improvement of care of the patients suffering from conditions, involving gangrene and tissue necrosis, which constitute the very purpose of this collective work.

Alexander A. Vitin, MD, Ph.D.
University of Washington
USA

Part 1

Fournier's Gangrene: Current Concepts and Treatment Options

1

Gangrene: The Prognostic Factors and Validation of Severity Index in Fournier's Gangrene

Ik Yong Kim
Department of Surgery, Yonsei University Wonju College of Medicine, Wonju, Korea

1. Introduction

Fournier's gangrene (FG) is a fulminant and life-threatening disease characterized by necrotizing fascitis of the perineal and genitourinary area resulting from polymicrobial infection. The polymicrobial organisms cause ascending reactions, activating various proteins and enzymes, leading to platelet aggregation, intravascular coagulation, tissue ischemic tissue change. This disease rapidly progresses, causing thrombosis and irreversible necrosis.

Most of patients had predisposed or concomitant diseases such as diabetes mellitus, alcoholism, hepatic diseases, renal diseases, and cardiac diseases.

It is a surgical emergency and requires prompt surgical debridement in most cases. For the treatment of Fournier's gangrene, aggressive wide necrotic tissue debridement for survival and the proper use of antibiotics, post-operative wound management, and proper reconstruction are required.

High mortality rates in Fournier's gangrene range from 6.3 to 50%, which indicates that the variable outcome of patients with the disease is multifactorial. In general, disease related factors and host-related factors are important prognostic factors.

To investigate clinical features and prognostic factors in patients who underwent the treatments of Fournier's gangrene, Acute Physiology and Chronic Health Evaluation (APACHE) II, and the Fournier's Gangrene Severity Index (FGSI) score which was first reported by Laor et al in 1995 were used and other scoring system. Among them, the FGSI is very useful and it can predict mortality and survival with a high probability for patients with Fournier's gangrene according to many authors. The quantification of the extent of the disease may help determine the outcome more precisely predictions for patients with Fournier's gangrene.

We analyzed 27 patients who underwent treatments due to Fournier's gangrene in our institution and evaluated predictive factors for mortality and survival based on pathogenesis, causative factors, and the subjects of progression. The result of this study showed that sepsis and FGSI of nine points or over at the time of hospitalization were significant risk factors for mortality.

2. History and pathophysiology of Fournier gangrene

2.1 History

Fournier's gangrene was first described by Jean Alfred Fournier (1832-1914) in 1883, a French dermatology/venereologist, a series in which previously healthy young men. He used the term-'**fulminant gangrene**-sudden onset necrotizing disease, rapid progression to gangrene and absence of a definite cause' of the penis and scrotum and his description was based on five young men with scrotal gangrene. Although this disease has been still called Fournier's gangrene to date, its concept has been changed and its causes have been identified in most cases. This condition is described as infective necrotizing fascitis which occurs in perineal, perianal, and genitourinary areas due to polymicrobial organisms regardless of gender and age.

Since Fournier's gangrene was first described, various changes have been made in the definition of the disease and its treatment methods.

2.2 Pathophysiology

Localized infection adjacent to a portal of entry is the inciting event in the development of Fournier gangrene. The polymicrobial organisms cause ascending reactions, activating various proteins and enzymes, leading to platelet aggregation, intravascular coagulation, tissue ischemic change. This disease rapidly progresses, causing thrombosis and irreversible necrosis in perineal and genitourinary areas.

It has been revealed that Fournier gangrene is a polymicrobial infection with an average of 2~4 isolates per case at wound cultures from patients. The bacteria involved act synergistically, via collagenases, hyaluronidases, and other enzymes to invade and destroy fascial planes

Ultimately, an obliterative endarteritis develops, and the ensuing cutaneous and subcutaneous vascular necrosis leads to localized ischemia and further bacterial proliferation. Rates of fascial destruction as high as 2-3 cm/h have been described in some reports. Infection of superficial perineal fascia (Colles fascia) may spread to the penis and scrotum via Buck and Dartos fascia, or to the anterior abdominal wall via Scarpa fascia, or vice versa. Perineal fascia is attached to the perineal body and urogenital diaphragm posteriorly and to the pubic rami laterally, thus limiting progression in these directions. Testicular involvement is rare, as the testicular arteries originate directly from the aorta and thus have a blood supply separate from the affected region.

2.3 Outcome/prognosis

Despite the development of modern intensive care and medical therapy, mortality rate from Fournier gangrene remains still high. The mortality rate for Fournier gangrene widely varies from 30 to 50%.

Prognosis may be affected by various factos, that include disease-related and host-related ones. The outcome of patients with the disease is indicated multifactorial.

Factors associated with high mortality include an anorectal source, advanced age, extensive disease (involving abdominal wall or thighs), shock or sepsis at presentation, renal failure, and hepatic dysfunction. Death usually results from systemic illness, such as sepsis, coagulopathy, acute renal failure, diabetic ketoacidosis, or multiple organ failure.

Most studies were conducted to investigate clinical features and prognostic factors in patients who underwent the treatments of Fournier's gangrene at a single institution. Progression to single-organ or multiorgan failure (MOF, MODF) may occur, usually as a result of gram-negative sepsis and is typically the cause of death. (Include acute renal failure and adult respiratory distress syndrome).

After recovering from a threatening condition, large scrotal, perineal, penile, and abdominal wall skin defects may require reconstructive procedures. Fatal tetanus associated with Fournier gangrene has been reported in the literature.

3. Clinical feature

3.1 Frequency

Fournier gangrene is relatively uncommon. The true incidence of the disease is unknown. A retrospective case review revealed 1726 cases documented in the literature from 1950 to 1999. An average of 97 cases per year was reported from 1989 to 1998. Poor socioeconomic conditions contribute to development of Fournier's Gangrene. However, regional prevalence and Ethnicity were not identified as relevant factors.

3.2 Age and sex

Mostly male-to-female ratio is mostly approximately 10:1 in large series. Rare reports including women, especially with postpartum perineal necrotizing fasciitis, but, the lower incidence in females may be caused by better drainage of the perineal region through vaginal secretions. Homosexual men may be at a higher risk of contracting Fournier gangrene; especially for infections caused by community-associated methicillin-resistant *Staphylococcus aureus* (MRSA).

Most cases occur in patients aged 30-60 years. When Fournier's gangrene was first described by Alfred Fournier, 'young age and male gender'were identified. The reported age of patients with the disease has progressively increased in the published data. In 1945, It was reported an average age of 40.9 years was reporeted; in 1979, Jones reported 51.3 years; Laor and colleagues reported an average age of 61 years old. In our analysis, we found an almost identical average of 57.3 years.

In our study, the male subjects composed 25 cases (92.6%) and the mean age of the subjects was 52.8 years. The age bracket of patients with Fournier's gangrene has commonly been found to be between 30 and 60 years. In this study, the mean age was 52.8 years and the patients with an age of less than 65 years accounted for 70.4 % of all subjects.

Regarding determinants of survival in older FG patients, it is now known that older patients have a lower survival rate. Clayton *et al.* statistically found that patients who survived were younger statistically than those who died of Fournier's gangrene (52 and 69 years old, respectively). Yilmazlar et al calculated a threshold age of 60 years in the ROC analysis (area under ROC curve: 0.709, 95%CI: 38.5–81.8). Logistic regression analysis identified age as an independent risk factor for mortality in large patients with Fournier's gangrene.

3.3 Predisposition to disease

Many predisposing factors have been reported, including systemic disease such as diabetes mellitus, alcoholism, chronic renal failure, chronic steroid use, malnutrition, HIV infection, and malignancy in FG. Any condition with decreased cellular immunity may predispose to the development of Fournier gangrene theoretically.

In our series, the concomitant diseases included diabetes mellitus in 29.6%; liver cirrhosis and alcoholic liver disease in 14.8% in our study. Diabetes mellitus was the most common comorbidity associated with FG and was present in 50% (24-72) of patients at the time of admission. **Table 1**

		No of Cases	Mean Age (yrs)	Gender	Origin		Fecal diversion (%)	DM (%)	Mortality (%)	FGSI *	
				M:F	Anorectal (%)	Urogenital (%)				Survival	Mortality
Laor et al	*1995*	30	61.0	NA	16.7	20.0	10.0	30.0	43.3	**6.9 ± 0.9**	**13.5 ± 1.5**
Villanueva-Saenz et al	*2002*	28	57.8	28	89.3	10.7	50.0	64.3	35.7		
Baek et al	*2003*	16	62.0	14:2	75.0	18.8	75.0	62.5	6.3		
Korkut et al	*2003*	45	54.6	NA	57.8	13.3	40.0	55.6	20.0		
Yeniyol et al	*2004*	25	51.7	NA	0.0	0.0	4.0	72.0	24.0	**3.0 ±1.8**	**12.0± 2.4**
Kim SK et al	*2006*	11	60.0	8:3	36.4	0.0	36.4	NA	27.3		
Yanar H et al	*2006*	35	58.6	25:10	17.1	8.6	14.3	45.7	40.0		
Basoglu et al	*2007*	45	54.0	44:1	48.9	2.0	46.7	24.4	8.9		
Corcoran et al	*2008*	68	55.8	54:14	38.2	11.8	26.5	52.9	10.3	**5.1± 3.4**	**10± 4.5**
Erol et al	*2009*	18	57.0	NA	NA	NA	22.2	55.6	22.2	**5.0± 2.9**	**13.5± 2.6**
Yilmazlar et al	*2010*	80	57.0	57:23	40.0	56.3	22.5	57.5	21.3	**4**	**14**
Kim KM et al	***2010***	27	52.8	25:2	59.3	40.7	51.9	29.6	14.8	**4.7± 0.4**	**9.3± 3.2**
mean		35.7	57.3		39.9	15.2	33.3	50.0	22.8	**4.0**	**14.0**

*Fournier's gangrene severity index

Table 1. Clinical feature and Outcome in patients with Fournier's gangrene

Diabetes has always been associated with an increased incidence of FG. Many authors reported the prevalence of diabetes as 50~73 percent, respectively. The high incidence of diabetics in FG was explained by the increased propensity to tissue ischemia caused by small-vessel disease. On the other hand, diabetes is associated with worse outcome and increased mortality, which could be explained by mutifactorial immunological system dysfunction, that included decreased phagocytosis ability, neutrophil dysfunction.

Although this association of unfavorable outcome and underlying diabetes has previously been mentioned, numerous review articles have failed to demonstrate a statistically significant difference.

One of the 15 nondiabetic patients died; however, the mortality rate among diabetics was higher (3 of 12 patients, 25 percent).

For pathogenesis, anorectal diseases were the most frequent causes of the infection.

In our retrospective review of 27 consecutive patients treated for FG at a single institution, factors such as the presence of sepsis, high FGSI and the initial surgical intervention affected outcome in univariate analyses.

The concomitant diseases of Fournier's gangrene have been known to include diabetes mellitus, alcoholism, chronic liver disease, various cancers, and immune suppression.

In this study, diabetes mellitus was found in eight patients; liver cirrhosis and alcoholic liver disease in four patients; and hypertension in nine patients. Bed ridden status due to paraplegia was also found in some patients.

3.4 Causative factors

Anorectal, genitourinary, and dermatologic sources are implicated in the pathogenesis of the disease. Localized infection adjacent to a portal of entry is often the inciting event in the development of Fournier gangrene. **Table 2.**

In men, anal intercourse may increase risk of perineal infection, either from blunt trauma to the area or by spread of anorectal microbes.

In women, septic abortions, hysterectomy, and episiotomy, vulvar or Bartholin gland abscesses are also documented sources.

Poor perineal hygiene or the presence of chronically indwelling catheters, such as in paraplegic patients, poses an increased risk in box sex.

Anorectal
- Trauma
- Ischiorectal, perirectal, or perianal abscesses
- Perianal fistulotomy
- Anal fissures; colonic perforations
- steroid enemas for radiation proctitis
- Rectal cancer

Genito urinary
- Trauma
- Urethral strictures with urinary extravasation
- Urethral catheterization or instrumentation, penile implants
- Periurethral infection ; chronic urinary tract infections;
- Epididymitis or orchitis
- Penile artificial implant, Foreign body

Hemipelvectomy
Cancer invasion to external genitalia
Septic abortion
Bartholin's duct abscess
Episiotomy

Dermatologic sources

Scrotal furuncle
Genital toilet (scrotum)
Blunt perineal trauma ; intramuscular injections, genital piercings
Perineal or pelvic surgery / Inguinal herniography

Idiopathic; more than 75%

Table 2. Causative Factors in Patients With Fournier's Gangrene

3.5 Clinical presentation

In general, most patients were reported to visit hospitals due to itching or discomfort of the external genitals. It was reported to take approximately 5 days from symptom expression to visiting the hospital. In this study, most patients suffered from perianal/scrotal swelling and pain as a main symptom. In addition, fever and chill, perianal/scrotal necrosis, purulent discharge, and voiding difficulty were also accompanied. The mean duration from the initiation of symptom expression to visiting the hospital was 99.8 hours, i.e. 4-5 days. When the patients were divided into anorectal and genitourinary groups and the characteristics of the subject groups were compared, no significant difference except for fecal diversion was found between the two groups. For anorectal diseases, fecal diversion is thought to be frequently conducted as wound management was difficult due to fecal contamination and the surgery site was perianal area.

All patients had at least one of the following early symptoms or signs: perianal or perineal pain, hyperemia, and fever.

The clinical presentation of the disease starts with a prodromal period of genital discomfort or pruritus, followed by genital erythema, swelling, crepitation and revealing subcutaneous gas formation.

Skin overlying the affected region may be normal, erythematous, edematous, cyanotic, bronzed, indurated, blistered, and/or frankly gangrenous in progression.

However, skin appearance often underestimates the degree of underlying disease. A feculent odor may be present secondary to infection with anaerobic bacteria. The gangrenous process will lead to drainage of the affected areas and demarcation between viable and dead tissue. The extent of the involved area may reach the abdominal wall, axilla, and thighs.

Crepitus may be present, but its absence does not exclude the presence of *Clostridium* species or other gas-producing organisms. Systemic symptoms (eg, fever, tachycardia, and hypotension) may be present.

In Fournier gangrene, obtain a thorough review of systems, including history of diabetes, alcohol abuse, cancer, colorectal or urogenital disease or surgery, steroid use, sexual history, and HIV status.

Sepsis at presentation was found in seven cases (25.9%). The mean duration from the expression of the symptoms to visiting the hospital was 99 hours.

3.6 Bacteriology

Both anaerobic and aerobic organisms isolated from wound cultures have been cited as an important bacteriologic principle in Fournier's gangrene. Paty and Smith found *E. coli, Bacteroides,* and streptococci to be the most common organisms.

Laor *et al.* determined the most common organisms were *E. coli* and *Streptococcus* species, with *Staphylococcus* and *Enterococcus* more commonly isolated than *Bacteroides.*

The mean microbial number of two was identified in microbial culture tests. *Streptococcus. species* was the most common microbial organism, accounting for 48.1%. *Enterococcus* and *Escherichia Coli* were found in 29.6% and 25.9%, respectively in our study. **Table 3.**

Bacterial organism	%
Streptococcus. Species	48.1
Enterococcus	29.6
Escherichia Coli	25.9
Unspecified G(+) rods	25.9
Klebsiela pneumoniae	18.5
Unspecified G(-) rods	14.8
Bacteroides species	1.1
Unspecified G(+) cocci	11.1
Coagulase-negative staphylococcus	7.4
Enterobacter species	7.4
Acinetobacter	3.7
Candida albicans	3.7

Table 3. Causative Bacterial organism of FG

The mean numbers of isolated microorganism per patient was reported to be four, and *Escherichia Coli* and Bacteroides were reported to be the most common microbes. In addition, Proteus, Staphylococcus, Pseudomonas, and Klabsiella were also reported. According to the results of this study, one to three microbes were identified. *Streptococcus species* and *Enterococcus* were common microbes, and Klebsilla and Bacteroides were also commonly identified as shown in previous study results.

Wound culture results from our series were similar to prior reported results with predominantly polymicrobial infections. It reveals a polymicrobial infection with an average of 4 isolates per case. *Streptococcus* species is the predominant aerobe, and *Bacteroides* is the predominant anaerobe.

Other microflora includes *Proteus, Staphylococcus, Enterococcus,* aerobic and anaerobic *Streptococcus, Pseudomonas, Klebsiella,* and *Clostridium.* Incidence of methicillin-resistant *Staphylococcus aureus* (MRSA) may be increase in being mentioned in literature

FG has always been considered a surgical emergency. Some articles have so far highlighted the poor prognosis of FG in patients with a delay in presentation and treatment.
In most studies the course of these patients was characterized by a more advanced disease necessitating more aggressive debridement with fecal diversion.
There are limitations in the design and interpretation of this study. First, we still have relatively few cases that were treated during a long period. Second, the retrospective study, the extent of the disease in terms of surface area and other prognostic variables were not included.

4. Differential diagnoses

- Balanitis, Epididymitis, Orchitis
- Testicular Torsion
- Hernias, Hydrocele
- Cellulitis, Gas Gangrene and
- Necrotizing Fasciitis

Cellulitis is used to indicate a nonnecrotizing inflammation of the skin and subcutaneous tissues, a process related to acute infection that does not involve the fascia or muscles. Cellulitis was classically considered to be an infection without formation of abscess and without purulent drainage or ulceration.
Gas gangrene, a subset of necrotizing myositis, is an emergent infectious disease. Organisms in the spore-forming clostridial species, including *Clostridium perfringens, Clostridium septicum,* and *Clostridium novyi,* cause most of the cases. A nonclostridial form is caused by a mixed infection of aerobic and anaerobic organisms. Disease has rapid onset of myonecrosis with muscle swelling, severe pain, gas production, and sepsis.
For more than a century, many authors have described soft tissue infections. Their occurrence has been on the rise because of an increase in immunocompromised patients with diabetes mellitus, cancer, alcoholism, vascular insufficiencies, organ transplants, HIV, or neutropenia.
Necrotizing fasciitis can occur after trauma or around foreign bodies in surgical wounds, or it can be idiopathic, as in scrotal or penile necrotizing fasciitis.
Necrotizing fasciitis has also been referred to as hemolytic streptococcal gangrene, Meleney ulcer, acute dermal gangrene, hospital gangrene, suppurative fascitis, and synergistic necrotizing cellulitis. Fournier gangrene is a form of necrotizing fasciitis that is localized to the scrotum and perineal area.
Necrotizing fasciitis is a progressive, rapidly spreading, inflammatory infection located in the deep fascia, with secondary necrosis of the subcutaneous tissues. Because of the presence of gas-forming organisms, subcutaneous air is classically described in necrotizing fasciitis. The speed of spread is directly proportional to the thickness of the subcutaneous layer. Necrotizing fasciitis moves along the deep fascial plane, rapidly progress. They require aggressive treatment to combat the associated high morbidity and mortality.

5. Diagnostic methods

5.1 Laboratory studies

The following studies are indicated in patients Fournier gangrene:

- CBC with differential count

- Electrolytes, BUN, creatinine, blood glucose levels: Acidosis with hyperglycemia or hypoglycemia may be present. Dehydration occurs as the disease progresses.
- ABG sampling to provide a more accurate assessment of acid/base disturbance
- Blood and urine cultures
- Disseminated intravascular coagulation (DIC) panel (coagulation studies, fibrinogen/fibrin degradation product levels) to find evidence of severe sepsis
- Cultures of any open wound or abscess

5.2 Imaging studies Fournier gangrene

Diagnosis of Fournier gangrene is primarily is based on clinical findings. Sensitivities and specificities of different radiologic modalities are not established.

Conventional radiography

Conventional radiography may demonstrate soft-tissue gas collections (manifest as areas of hyperlucency), even4 before they are clinically apparent. Scrotal tissue edema may be observed on radiographs. Absence of air on plain films does not exclude the diagnosis.

Ultrasonography

Ultrasonography may reveal other causes of acute scrotal pain, including intratesticular injury, scrotal cellulitis, epididymoorchitis, testicular torsion, and inguinal hernia.
Gas in the scrotal wall is the "sonographic hallmark" of Fournier gangrene. Air may be appreciated in perineal and/or perirectal areas. Scrotal wall edema may be seen. Testes and epididymides are usually normal.

Computerized tomography

Findings include soft-tissue and fascial thickening, fat stranding, and soft-tissue gas collections. CT scans defines the extent of the disease more specifically. CT scan often identifies the underlying cause of the infection (eg, perirectal abscess). This modality may assist in surgical planning.

MRI

MRI use is not well described in the literature. MRI may define soft-tissue pathology more distinctly than CT scan but should not delay operative intervention if the diagnosis is highly suspected.

6. Treatment & management

6.1 Resuscitation & early care

The following treatment is indicated in patients with Fournier gangrene:

- Initially, aggressive resuscitation in anticipation of surgery - Airway management if indicated, crystalloid replacement if dehydrated or displaying signs of shock
- Supplemental oxygen, intravenous (IV) access, and continuous cardiac monitoring

Early, broad-spectrum antibiotics are indicated, including the following:

- Ampicillin/sulbactam
- Ticarcillin/clavulanate
- Piperacillin/tazobactam
- Penicillinase-resistant penicillin, aminoglycoside, and metronidazole or clindamycin
- Coverage for methicillin-resistant *Staphylococcus aureus* (MRSA), such as vancomycin

Tetanus prophylaxis is indicated if soft-tissue injury is present.
Irrigation with superoxidized water and packing with gauze soaked with zinc peroxide and hydrogen peroxide may be helpful.
Surgical consultation is imperative. Immediate urologic, colorectal consultation is mandatory.

6.2 Medication summary

The goals of pharmacotherapy in Fournier gangrene are to reduce morbidity and to control the infection.

Antibiotics

Initiate early broad-spectrum antibiotics as soon as possible. Providing coverage for gram-positive, gram-negative, aerobic, and anaerobic bacteria is essential. Penicillins and beta-lactamase inhibitors or triple antibiotics are potential choices.

Vancomycin

Ampicillin-sulbactam sodium

Ticarcillin and clavulanate potassium

Piperacillin/tazobactam

Gentamicin

Metronidazole

Clindamycin

6.3 Immunizations

Patients with fatal tetanus associated with Fournier gangrene have been documented in literatures. Patients with noncurrent tetanus status require immunization in the emergency department.

Diphtheria and tetanus toxoid (Decavac)

Tetanus toxoid is manufactured by first culturing *Clostridium tetani* and then detoxifying the toxin with formaldehyde. This toxoid is commonly combined with diphtheria toxoid, and both serve to induce production of serum antibodies to toxins produced by the bacteria.

6.4 Surgical management

Aggressive surgical debridement may have a positive effect on survival. Although Clayton *et al.* and Laor *et al.* suggested that the extent of disease was not predictive of outcome, Spirnak *et al.* associated the greater mortality rate for patients who underwent more frequent operations to the presence of a greater extent of the disease. Others found that the extent of body surface area involved in the necrotizing process was directly related to mortality.
Surgeon or urologist may order further diagnostic tests in patients with Fournier gangrene, including cystourethroscopy, retrograde urethrography, sigmoidoscopy, barium enema, tissue biopsy, and examination under anesthesia.
Urinary and/or fecal diversion (eg, suprapubic catheterization, ileostomy or colostomy) may be required depending on the source of infection.[5]

If the initial facility does not have the capability to provide operative therapy in a timely fashion, arrange for **transfer** once the patient has been stabilized and resuscitative efforts have begun. Patients often require a multidisciplinary team, including urologist, general surgeon, and team for intensive care. Transfer to a tertiary facility may be required if these resources are not available at the initial facility.

Multiple surgical debridements in the operating room may be required to effectively remove all necrotic tissue. Patients with Fournier gangrene undergo an average of 2-4 operative procedures during their initial hospitalization. In our study, 17 cases (63%), required surgical treatments of fecal or urinary diversion. Orchiectomy and/or penectomy are rarely required.

Reconstructive surgery due to wide wound defects was required in 11 cases (40.7%). The mean length of stay in hospital was 70.8 days.

Hyperbaric oxygen therapy (HBO) has been used as an adjuvant to surgical and antimicrobial therapy, especially in patients for whom conventional treatment failed, in those with documented clostridial involvement, or in those with myonecrosis or deep tissue involvement. HBO is postulated to reduce systemic toxicity, prevent extension of necrotizing infection, and inhibit growth of anaerobic bacteria. However, in one series, there was actually a trend toward increased mortality in patients undergoing HBO therapy. Decisions regarding hyperbaric therapy must be made on an individual basis and should be an adjuvant to debridement and antimicrobial therapy.

7. Outcome and prognosis

There is no consensus on which clinical variables predict a poor outcome in FG. Retrospective studies have implicated increasing age, diabetes mellitus, delay in presentation / treatment and extent of involvement (BSA, Body Surface area). While BSA was suggestive of a poor prognosis of all the operative characteristics examined, only lower extremity or abdominal wall involvement was associated with inpatient mortality.

Previous reports suggest that older, debilitated or bedridden patients with multiple comorbidities presenting with advanced FG are more likely to have poor outcomes. Factors associated with an improved prognosis include age younger than 60 years, localized clinical disease, absence of systemic toxicity, and sterile blood cultures.

Four patients (14.8%) died during the treatment; three patients due to sepsis and one patient who had scrotal abscess accompanied with incarcerated inguinal hernia died due to renal failure. However, our results indicate that with, age, comorbidity, use of early aggressive therapy and time to presentation do not affect prognosis.

For host related factors, the novel scoring system should be validated through other prospective studies and independent observations and can be applied in clinical practice

The number of patients with FG is significant and the mortality ranges between 15 to 50%, showing various prognoses. Higher mortality was reported to be seen in the cases of anal diseases, the elderly, diabetes mellitus, invasion to the abdominal wall and the thigh, higher FGSI, shock and sepsis at the time of hospitalization, and accompanying hepatic failure and renal failure.

The FGSI was developed to help clinicians predict outcome in patients with FG. **Table 4**. A score of 0-4 is assigned to each of the following parameters: temperature; heart rate; respiratory rate; serum sodium, potassium, bicarbonate, and creatinine levels; hematocrit; and WBC count. Its modified scoring system also has been developed, which has been shown to aid in prognosis. **Table 5.**

	High Abnormal Values				Normal	Low Abnormal Values			
Physiologic Variables / Point assignment	+4	+3	+2	+1	0	+1	+2	+3	+4
Temperature (C) [	>41	39–40.9	–	38.5–38.9	36–38.4	34–35.9	32–33.9	30–31.9	<29.9
Heart rate (bpm)	>180	140–179	110–139	–	70–109	–	55–69	40–54	<39
Respiratory rate	>50	35–49	–	25–34	12–24	10–11	6–9	–	<5
Serum potassium (mmol/L)	>7	6–6.9	–	5.5–5.9	3.5–5.4	3–3.4	2.5–2.9	–	<2.5
Serum sodium (mmol/L)	>180	160–179	155–159	150–154	130–149	–	120–129	110–119	<110
Serum creatinine (mg/100 ml) (x2 for acute renal failure)	>3.5	2-3.4	1.5-1.9	–	0.6-1.4	–	<0.6	–	–
Hematocrit (%)	>60	–	50–59	46–49	30–45	–	20–29	–	<20
White blood count (91000/mm3)	>40	–	20–39.9	15–19.9	3–14.9	–	1–2.9	–	<1
Serum bicarbonate, (venous) (mmol/L)	>52	41–51	–	32–40	22–31	–	18–21	15–17	<15

Table 4. Fournier's gangrene severity index

Laor et al reported that a FGSI score greater than 9 indicated a 75% probability of mortality while a score of 9 or less was associated with a 78% probability of survival. This cutoff point has subsequently been validated in other small retrospective series. However, Tuncel et al of 20 men with FG demonstrated no association between FGSI and mortality, and stated that specific metabolic parameters (serum albumin and alkaline phosphatase), predisposing factors and disease extent should be assessed together to predict treatment outcome and survival.

In our study, the mean FGSI was 9.25 in patients who had died and 4.69 in patients who survived. Of the factors affecting the mortality, sepsis and FGSI of 9 points or over at the time of hospitalization were statistically significant. **Table 6.**

The morbidity of FG has been gradually increasing and its causal diseases and causal microbes have also varied. For the treatment of Fournier's gangrene, active wound managements such as early diagnosis, wide excision for necrotic tissue, the proper use of antimicrobials, and continuous postoperative aseptic dressing are required.

Variables	+4	+3	+2	+1	0	+1	+2	+3	+4
a. Physiological parameters									
Temperature (C) [	>41	39–40.9	–	38.5–38.9	36–38.4	34–35.9	32–33.9	30–31.9	<29.9
Heart rate	>180	140–179	110–139	–	70–109	–	55–69	40–54	<39
Respiratory rate	>50	35–49	–	25–34	12–24	10–11	6–9	–	<5
Serum potassium (mmol/L)	>7	6–6.9	–	5.5–5.9	3.5–5.4	3–3.4	2.5–2.9	–	<2.5
Serum sodium (mmol/L)	>180	160–179	155–159	150–154	130–149	–	120–129	110–119	<110
Serum creatinine (mg/100 ml) (x2 for acute renal failure)	>3.5	2-3.4	1.5-1.9	–	.6-1.4	–	<0.6	–	–
Hematocrit (%)	>60	–	50–59	46–49	30–45	–	20–29	–	<20
White blood count (91000/mm3)	>40	–	20–39.9	15–19.9	3–14.9	–	1–2.9	–	<1
Serum bicarbonate, (venous) (mmol/L)	>52	41–51	–	32–40	22–31	–	18–21	15–17	<15

b. Dissemination score

Fournier's gangrene confined to the urogenital and/or anorectal region, add "1"

Fournier's gangrene confined to the pelvic region, add "2"

Fournier's gangrene extending beyond the pelvic region, add "6"

c. Age score

Age ≥60 years, add "1"

Age <60 years, add "1"

UFGSI = A+B+C

Table 5. The Uludag Fournier's gangrene severity index Yilmazlar T et al (2007)

		Total N=27	Mortality N=4(%),	Odds ratio(95%, CI)	p
Age (years)	<65	19	3 (15.8)	0.762 (0.067-8.665)	1.000
	≥65	8	1 (12.5)		
Duration	<48 hours	9	1 (11.1)	1.600(0.142-18.000)	1.000
of symptoms	>48 hours	18	3(16.7)		
Infection source	Anorectal	16	2 (12.5)	1.556 (0.185-13.108)	1.000
	Genitourinary	11	2 (18.2)		
Sepsis	Present	7	3 (42.9)	14.250 (1.162-174.801)	*0.042*
	Absent	20	1 (5.0)		
FGSI*	≤9	24	2 (8.3)	22.000(1.334-362.916)	*0.049*
	>9	3	2 (66.7)		
DM or Liver	Present	12	3 (25.0)	4.667 (0.418-52.121)	0.294
disease	Absent	15	1 (6.7)		
No of	<2	9	3 (33.3)	0.118 (0.010-1.359)	0.093
Debridement	≥2	18	1 (5.6)		
Diversion	Performed	17	2 (11.8)	0.533 (0.063-4.531)	0.613
	Not performed	10	2 (20.0)		

*FGSI, Fourier's gangrene severity index

Table 6. Prognostic factors for mortality of Fournier's gangrene *Kim KM et al 2010*

	Survival vs. Nonsurvival (N)	p	References
Age (years)	63 vs. 17	*0.002*	*Yilmazlar et al 2010*
FGSI(median)		*<0.001*	
Extent of the disease (Grade I,II, III)		*<0.001*	
Need for ICU		*<0.001*	
Need for Ventilator		*<0.001*	
Length of Hospital stay (days, median)		*0.002*	
RR	14 vs. 4	*0.003*	*Erol et al 2009*
Tempaerature		*0.046*	
Median BSA*		*0.018*	
Charlson Comorbidity Index		*0.008*	
Life expectancy for 10 y (%)		*0.008*	
RR	61 vs. 7	*0.021*	*Corcoran et al 2008*
Serum bicarbonate		*0.001*	
FGSI		*0.006*	
Serum lactate		*0.001*	
Serum calcium		*0.032*	
Time to consult	19 vs. 6	*0.002*	*Yeniyol et al 2004*
BSA		*0.0001*	
FGSI		*0.0001*	
Sepsis	23 vs. 4	*0.042*	*Kim et al 2010*
FGSI* ≤9 vs. >9		*0.049*	

BSA _ body surface area.

Table 7. Prognostic factors for mortality of Fournier's gangrene

Aggressive and early surgical débridement continues to be the mainstay of treatment of FG in most series. It was reported that the number of operative débridements negatively affects survival, speculating that patients requiring multiple débridements had greater extent of disease, were less healthy at baseline and had progressed to systemic sepsis despite aggressive surgical therapy. Factors confounding the significance of the number of débridement necessary for disease control among survivors include total surface area involved, variation in the extent of the initial resection and whether the patient is healthy enough to survive multiple procedures

The result of our study showed that sepsis and FGSI of nine points or over at the time of hospitalization were statistically significant as factors affecting mortality. The patients included in the aforementioned criteria could show poor prognoses such as DIC, acute renal failure, acute renal failure, and multiorgan failure.

If necessary, hyperbaric oxygen therapy can be helpful, and furthermore, reconstruction surgery may be necessary later.

In this study, FG was investigated in relatively many cases at a single institution compared to other studies conducted in Korea. Further studies with a larger subject population will be required.

8. Conclusion

Despite the development of modern intensive care and medical therapy, Fournier's gangrene remains a fulminant and life-threatening disease, mortality rates have improved as a result of advances in surgical and critical care. Early diagnosis and surgical treatment of Fournier's gangrene are required.

Comprehensive evaluation of metabolic and physiological parameters, predisposing factors, and the extent of disease are also essential for early diagnosis and treatment.

There is no current consensus regarding the use of individual patient admission characteristics or laboratory values as prognostic indicator, sepsis at presentation and lower extremity/abdominal wall involvement were associated with disease severity and inpatient mortality in large series.

The FGSI remains a simple method of assessing severity of presentation and predicting outcome in this complex patient population.

Poor prognoses were seen in the cases of sepsis and FGSI of nine points or over at the time of hospitalization. Our results support previous findings that a FGSI threshold of 9 is a sensitive and specific predictor of mortality during initial assessment. Therefore, the careful observation of vital signs and active treatments are required to treat Fournier's gangrene.

9. References

Ayan F, Sunamak O, Paksoy SM et al (2005) Fournier's gangrene: a retrospective clinical study on forty-one patients. ANZ J Surg 75:1055–1058

Baek JH, Yoon SJ, Oh JH. (2003) Surgical management of Fournier's gangrene.J Korean Soc Coloproctol 19:349-53.

Baskin LS, Carroll PR, Cattolica EV, et al. (1990) Necrotising soft tissue infections of the perineum and genitalia: bacteriology, treatment and risk assessment. *Br J Urol.* 65:524-529.

Basoglu M, Ozbey I, Atamanalp SS et al. (2007) Management of Fournier's gangrene: review of 45 cases. Surg Today 37:558–563

Clayton MD, Fowler JE, Sharifi R. (1990) Causes, presentation and survival of fifty-seven patients with necrotizing fasciitis of the male genitalia. *Surg Gynecol Obstet.* 170:49-53.

Corcoran AT, Smaldone MC, Gibbons EP, et al. (2008) Validation of the Fournier's gangrene severity index in a large contemporary series.*J Urol.* 180:944-948.

Eke N (2000) Fournier's gangrene: a review of 1726 cases. Br J Surg 87:718–728

Ersay A, Yilmaz G, Akgu¨n Y et al (2007) Factors affecting mortality of Fournier's gangrene: review of 70 patients. ANZ J Surg 77:43–48

Fournier JA. (1883) Gangrene foudroyante de la verge. Medecin Practique 4:589–97.

Kim KM, Seong SH, Won DY, Ryu H, Kim IY (2010) The Prognostic Factors and Severity Index in Fournier's Gangrene. J Korean Soc Coloproctol 26:29-33.

Kim SK, Park JI, Joo YT, Park ST, Ha WS, Hong SC, et al. (2006)Fournier's gangrene: clinical analysis of 11 patients. J Korean Surg Soc 71: 274-8.

Korkut M, Ic¸o¨z G, Dayangac¸ M et al (2003) Outcome analysis in patients with Fournier's gangrene: report of 45 cases. Dis Colon Rectum 46:649–652

Laor E, Palmer LS, Tolia BM, Reid RE, Winter HI (1995) Outcome prediction in patients with Fournier's gangrene. J Urol 154:89–92

Lin E, Yang S, Chiu AW et al (2005) Is Fournier's gangrene severity index useful for predicting outcome of Fournier's gangrene? Urol Int 75:119–122

Palmer LS, Winter HI, Tolia BM, Reid RE, Laor E (1995) The limited impact of involved surface area and surgical de´bridement on survival in Fournier's gangrene. Br J Urol 76:208–212

Quatan N, Kirby RS. (2004) Improving outcomes in Fournier's gangrene. *BJU Int.* 93:691.

Spirnak JP, Resnick MI, Hampel N. Fournier's gangrene: report of 20 patients. *J Urol.* 1984;131:289-292.

Tahmaz L, Erdemir F, Kibar Y et al (2006) Fournier's gangrene: report of thirty-three cases and a review of the literature. Int J Urol 13:960–967

Tuncel A, Aydin O, Tekdogan U et al (2006) Fournier's gangrene: three years of experience with 20 patients and validity of the Fournier's gangrene severity index score. Eur Urol 50:838- 843

Villanueva-Sa´enz E, Martinez Herna´ndez-Magro P, Valde´s Ovalle M et al (2002) Experience in management of Fournier's gangrene. Tech Coloproctol 6:5–10

Yanar H, Taviloglu K, Ertekin C et al (2006) Fournier's gangrene: risk factors and strategies for management. World J Surg 30:1750–1754

Yeniyol CO, Suelozgen T, Arslan M, Ayder AR (2004) Fournier's gangrene: experience with 25 patients and use of Fournier's gangrene severity index score. Urology 64:218–222

Yilmazlar T, Ozturk E, Alsoy A, Ozguc H (2007) Necrotizing soft tissue infections: APACHE II score, dissemination, and survival. World J Surg 31:1858–1862

2

Fournier's Gangrene: Diagnostic and Therapeutic Considerations

David Kearney
Cork University Hospital
Ireland

1. Introduction

Fournier's gangrene is a necrotising fasciitis of the genitalia. Jean Alfred Fournier (1832-1914) was the first French syphilologist, the first professor of cutaneous and syphilitic diseases at the Paris Faculty of Medicine, and the most prominent European venereologist of the second half of the 19th century. He first described idiopathic, rapily progressive necrotizing gangrene of the male genitalia in 1883 and emphasised three characteristics; abrupt onset of scrotal pain and swelling in a healthy young man, rapid progression to gangrene, and the absence of a definitive cause (Fournier, 1883). Fournier's original description included five otherwise healthy young males with scrotal gangrene and emphasised the sudden onset and rapid progression of the disease. Over the years several terms have been applied to Fournier's gangrene including 'streptococcus gangrene', 'necrotising fasciitis', 'periurethral phlegmon', 'phagedena' and 'synergistic necrotising cellulitis' (Eke, 2000). Although originally described in healthy young men Fournier's gangrene is frequently seen in elderly patients as well as children (Woodside, 1980) and women (Lowthian and Gillard Jr, 1980).

2. Pathophysiology

Initially described as an idiopathic entity, a source of infection can now be identified in the majority of cases. Perineal and genital skin infections comprise most of the sources identified but anorectal or urogenital trauma, diverticular disease, pelvic and perineal injury and pelvic intervetions are other causes of Fournier s gangrene (Thwaini et al., 2006). In a large case series by Eke the distribution of the source of sepsis was 24% dermatological, 21% colorectal, 19% urological and unknown in 34% of patients (Eke, 2000). Whilst this condition does continue to effect healthy young men, the mean age of patients is between 50-65 years of age. Most patients have associated co-morbidities such as diabetes, alcoholism or HIV infection (Kuo et al., 2007). Diabetes is reported to be present in 20%-70% of patients with Fournier's gangrene (Morpurgo, 2002) and chronic alcoholism in 25%-50% of cases (Clayton et al., 1990).

The disease is believed to be an obliterative end-arteritis caused by the spread of micro-organisms. Inflammation and oedema from infection results in an impaired local blood supply, leading to vascular thrombosis in the cutaneous and subcutaneous tissues. Peri-fascial dissection with subsequent spread of bacteria and progression to gangrene of the overlying tissues ensues (Levenson et al., 2008). The rate of fascial necrosis has been estimated to be as high as 3 cm per hour making early diagnosis crucial (Safioleas et al., 2006). The subcutaneous infection with oedema and inflammation in an enclosed space impairs the blood supply and the resulting hypoxia permits the growth of facultative and obligatory anaerobes. These anaerobic micro-organisms produce hydrogen and nitrogen that accumulate in subcutaneous tissues resulting in crepitus (Hejase et al., 1996). The presence of subcutaneous emphysema signifies anaerobic conditions in the affected area (Wolach et al., 1989). Deeper infection that extends below the facial layers to involve myonecrosis not generally thought to be a feature of classical Fournier's gangrene, although it has been described (Rye et al., 1987).

Testicular involvement is rare in Fournier's gangrene because of the separate blood supply to the testes (Gupta et al., 2007). In a retrospective review of 29 patients over a 13-year period Baskin et al. reported that only three patients underwent orchidectomy due to testicular gangrene (Baskin et al., 1990). Ayan et al reviewed 41 cases of Fournier's gangrene and found that a bilateral orchidectomy was performed in 4 patients and a unilateral orchidectomy was performed in 5 patients (Ayan et al., 2005). In his large review of 1726 patients Eke suggested that when testicular involvement does occur it indicates a retroperitoneal or intra-abdominal source of infection (Eke, 2000). Penis involvement is also rare and the corpora are usually spared while the skin sloughs off. Thrombosis of the corpus spongiosum and cavernosum has, however, been reported (Campos and Martos, 1990).

3. Bacteriology

There have been many types of bacteriological culture encountered in Fournier's gangrene, both single strain and polymicrobial culture. In their experience of 38 patients Hejase et al found that 90% of the patients grew polymicrobial flora, including gram-positive and gram-negative rods and gram-positive cocci. The main strains grown were Staphylococcus aureus, β-hemolytic Streptococcus, Pseudomonas sp., E. coli and Klebsiella sp. (Hejase et al., 1996). In 5% of their cases no growth was reported. Korkut et al had a 64% positive culture rate of the 36 patients in their case series who had cultures sent during their initial debridement, and the leading mircro-organism was Escherichia coli (Korkut et al., 2003). In their review of 70 patients with Fournier's gangrene Ersay et al found that the most frequent bacterial organisms cultured from the wounds were Escherichia coli (40.0%), Bacteroides spp. (38.6%), Streptococcus spp. (37.1%), Enterococcus spp. (27.1%), Staphylococcus spp. (25.7%), Pseudomonas spp. (24.3%), Klebsiella pneumoniae (20.0%), and Proteus spp. (18.6%). The bacterial organisms cultured from wound however were not independent predictors of outcome (Ersay et al., 2007). Kuo et al cutured a variety of oganisms in their series of 44 patients in northern Taiwan (Kuo et al., 2007). These were cultured from necrotic tissue or pus during surgery or at the bedside. Only 1 organism was identified in 13 patients whilst culture results in 28 patients demonstrated polymicrobial infection. In 3 patients wound cultures were negative. The most commonly isolated organisms from wound were Escherichia coli in 26 patients, Bacteroides fragilis in 17 patients, Klebsiella pneumoniae in 16 patients, Enterococcus spp. in 14 patients and Proteus mirabilis in 10 patients. Similar to the case series by Ersay et al, mortality was not related to the specific isolated organism. In their review of 43 reconstructive patients Ferreira et al had a positive culture from 35 of the 43 patients, with 29 (82.9%) of these being polymicrobial (Ferreira et al., 2007). The most common orgaisms isolated were Staphylococcus aureus (21 patients), Escherichia coli and Pseudomonas aeruginosa (11).

In their review article on Fornier's gangrene Thwaini et al state that "cultures from the wounds commonly show polymicrobial infections by aerobes and anaerobes, which include coliforms, klebsiella, streptococci, staphylococci, Clostridia, Bacteroides and Cornybacteria. On average, at least three organisms are cultured from each diagnosed patient" (Thwaini et al., 2006). Along with the above organisms mentioned there have been cases reported of Fournier's gangrene caused by unusual organisms such as Clostridium perfrinogens (Korhonen et al., 1998) and Clostridium tetani (Omotoso, 1990).

4. Clinical

The clinical features of Fournier's gangrene include sudden pain in the scrotum, prostration, pallor and pyrexia. At first only the scrotum is involved, but if unchecked, the cellulitis spreads until the entire scrotal coverings slough, leaving the testes exposed but healthy (Russell et al., 2000). The presentation may also be insidious as opposed to the classical sudden onset presentation. One overwhelming feature of the presentation is the strong 'repulsive, fetid odour' that is associated with the condition (Randall, 1920). Patients can present with varying signs and symptoms including fever greater than 38°C, scrotal swelling and erythema, purulence or wound discharge, crepitation or fluctulance (Ozden Yeniyol et al., 2004). In their case series Ferreira et al found that the most common presentations were scrotal swelling, fever and pain. The mean interval between initial symptoms and arrival at the hospital was 5.1 ± 3.1 days. Scrotal involvement was found in 93.3% of cases, the penis was involved in 46.5% of cases, and the perineum or peri-anal region was involved in 37.2% of cases (Ferreira et al., 2007). Ersay et al found that the most common presentation was peri-anal/scrotal pain (78.6%) followed by tachycardia (61.4%), purulent discharge from the perineum (60%), crepitus (54.3%) and fever (41.4%) (Ersay et al., 2007). Crepitus of the inflamed tissue is a common feature of the disease due to the presence of gas forming organisms. As the subcutaneous inflammation worsens, necrotic patches start appearing over the overlying skin and progress to extensive necrosis (Laucks 2nd, 1994). The spread if infection is along the facial planes and is usually limited by the attachment of the Colles' fascia in the perineum (Thwaini et al., 2006). Infection can spread to involve the scrotum, peinis and can spread up the anterior abdominal wall, up to the clavicle (Saijo et al., 1990). As mentioned previously testicular involvement is rare in Fournier's gangrene because of the separate blood supply to the testes, although it can occur and result in unilateral or bilateral orchidectomy.

5. Differential diagnosis

Although the diagnosis of Fournier's gangrene is usually obvious due to the gangrene, patients may present at an earlier stage with an acutely swollen tender scrotum. Differential diagnoses in this scenario include intra-testicular injuries such as fracture and haematoma, extra-testicular injuries including haematomas or hematoceles, torsion of the spermatic cord, haemmorhage and necrosis of a testicular tumour, strangulated scrotal hernia, and inflammatory disease (Begley et al., 1988). Aside from the rare abscess or granulomatous infection the majority of inflammatory diseases affecting the scrotum are epididymitis and epididymo-orchitis.

6. Investigations

The diagnosis of Fournier's gangrene is primarily clinical. Imaging modalities may be helpful in those where the presentation is atypical or when there is concern regarding the true extent of the disease (Thwaini et al., 2006). Ultrasound has been shown to be effective in demonstrating specific features of Fournier's gangrene, although CT has greater specificity for evaluating the disease. Unlike other conditions that cause acute scrotal pain, in Fournier's gangrene the scrotal contents- the testes and epididymides- are normal, and no masses or other abnormal structures are present. Instead the ultrasound characteristics of Fournier's gangrene include marked thickening of scrotal skin and, most significantly, air in the subcutaneous tissues. If the patient has more advanced disease, the skin thickening and subcutaneous air can be traced from the scrotum with ultrasound to demonstrate it's full extent (Begley et al., 1988). Because the majority of cases of Fournier's gangrene are not primary and are secondary to other conditions described earlier (e.g. diverticulitis), CT plays an important role in the diagnosis as well as the evaluation of disease extent for appropriate surgical treatment. In their review of the role of imaging in Fournier's gangrene, Levenson et al describe the CT features seen in the disease: "The CT features on Fournier's gangrene include soft-tissue thickening and inflammation. CT can demonstrate asymmetric fascial thickening, any co-existing fluid collection or abscess, fat stranding around involved structures, and subcutaneous emphysema secondary to gas-forming bacteria. The subcutaneous emphysema in Fournier's gangrene dissects along fascial planes and can extend from the scrotum and perineum to the inguinal regions, thighs, abdominal wall, and retroperitoneum. The underlying cause of Fournier's gangrene, such as perianal abscess, a fistulous tract, or an intra-abdominal or retroperitoneal infection process may also be demonstrated on CT. In cases caused by colonic perforation, not only does CT demonstrate extraluminal foci of air, but extravasation of enteric contrast material may also be seen" (Levenson et al., 2008). Features of Fournier's gangrene can also be seen on plain radiography with hyperlucencies representing soft-tissue gas seen overlying the scrotum or perineum. Subcutaneous emphysema may also be seen within the soft tissues. Deep fascial gas is rarely seen at plain film radiography, which represents a significant weakness of this modality in the diagnosis and evaluation of Fournier's gangrene (Wysoki et al., 1997).

Routine blood investigations should be sent including a FBC, urea & electrolytes, C-Reactive Protein (CRP), glucose, and Arterial Blood Gas (ABG). The LRINEC (Laboratory Risk Indicator for Necrotizing Fasciitis) is a robust laboratory measurement score capable of determining even clinically early cases of necrotizing fasciitis (Wong et al., 2004). Using logistic regression analysis of independent variables from 89 cases of necrotizing fasciitis 6 factors were identified to be independent predictors. A summary table of these variables is shown below in Table 1.

Of the cohort of 89 patients only 13 (14.6%) patients had a diagnosis or suspicion of necrotizing fasciitis on admission. A majority were therefore missed, resulting in delayed operative debridement. In contrast, 80 (89.9%) of these patients had a LRINEC score of ≥6. According to Wong et al the biochemical and hematologic changes in necrotizing fasciitis develop early in the evolution of the disease and the LRINEC score can stratify patients into high and moderate risk categories even when the clinical picture is still equivocal.

Laor et al determined outcome predition on 30 patients with Fournier's gangrene and proposed a Fourner's gangrene severity index (Laor et al., 1995). Admission laboratory parameters that were statistically related to outcome included hematocrit, blood urea

Variable, Units	Score
C-Reactive Protein, mg/L	
<150	0
≥150	4
Total white cell count, per mm^3	
<15	0
15-25	1
>25	2
Haemoglobin, g/dL	
>13.5	0
11-13.5	1
<11	2
Sodium, mmol/L	
≥135	0
<135	2
Creatanine, µmol/L	
≤141	0
>141	2
Glucose, mmol/L	
≤10	0
>10	1

Table 1. Summary of the Laboratory Risk Indicator for Necrotizing Fasciitis (LRINEC) score. A LRINEC score of ≥6 should raise the suspicion of necrotizing fasciitis among patients with severe soft tissue infections, and a score ≥8 is strongly predictive of this disease (Wong et al., 2004).

nitrogen, calcium, albumin, alkaline phospatase and cholesterol levels. White blood count, platelets, potassium, bicorbonate, blood urea nitrogen, total protein, albumen and lactic dehydrogenise levels one week following hospitalization were also associated with outcome. These levels combined with the acute physiology and chronic health evaluation II severity score was used to create the Fournier's gangrene severity index. The authors found that using a threshold of 9 on the severity index there was a 75% probability of death with a score greater than 9, while a score less than 9 was associated with a 78% probability of survival (p=0.008).

7. Treatment

The cornerstones of treatment of Fournier's gangrene are urgent surgical debridement of all necrotic tissue as well as high doses of broad-spectrum antibiotics. Urgent resuscitation with fluids as well as blood transfusions may be needed. Empirical broad spectrum antibiotics should be initiated regardless of the Gram-stain and culture results, and the antibiotics chosen should cover streptococci, staphylococci, gram-negative Coliforms, Pseudomonas, Bacteroides and Clostridia (Laucks II, 1994). Early surgical debridement is the primary aim of treatment and if delayed will have a negative impact on prognosis (Elliott et al., 2000).

The goal of surgery is to excise all non-viable tissue until well-perfused viable tissue is reached. The subcutaneous disease may be more extensive than the cutaneous involvement and more radial debridement may need to be undertaken than originally planned pre-operatively. Care must be taken not to open up deeper fascial planes that were not originally involved. Depending on the original foci of the disease, urinary or faecal diversion may be necessary. Multiple debridements of necrotic tissue are the rule rather than the exception. As mentioned previously, orchidectomy is a rare but sometimes necessary eventuality of extensive Fournier's gangrene.

Once the infection has subsided the scrotum has traditionally been left to heal by secondary intention as it has been noted to possess a remarkable ability to regenerate and heal (Thomas, 1956). The use of skin grafts and flaps are common to provide coverings of debrided tissue. In their review of 43 reconstructive cases Ferreira et al performed surgical debridement of scrotal, penile, and perineal necrosis along with other involved areas in all patients, including seven patients who required debridement twice, and one patient who required debridement three times (Ferreira et al., 2007). All patients received delayed surgical reconstruction after the appearance of healthy granulation tissue at the base of the wound. The mean time between the last debridement performed and the first reconstruction was 37.4 days. In total, 61 reconstructive procedures were performed in the 43 patients with up to four operations being performed on each patient. The superomedial thigh flap was performed for scrotum reconstruction in 26 patients. Split-thickness skin grafts were the major solution for covering penile skin losses. In four patients with urethral stricture, tubed urethroplasty was performed using free full-thickness skin grafts. Mean hospital stay was 73.6 ± 42.5 days.

Along with the increased use of skin flaps & grafts to cover bare areas after surgical debridement, the use of vacuum-assisted closure (VAC) has increased in popularity and aided the healing process in patients with Fournier's gangrene. In their case series of 35 patients with Fournier's gangrene who received surgical debridement of necrotic areas, Czymek et al compared patients who were treated with conventional dressings to those who received VAC dressings over an 11 year period (Czymek et al., 2009). In the conventional dressings group, patients had their dressings changed once per day until the wounds were clean and healthy and local wounds could be closed with meshed grafts or flaps. In the VAC therapy group the VAC dressing was initiated 3-5 days after primary debridement. Continuous negative pressure of 75 mmHg was applied to the wounds and the VAC was changed every 48 hours. Similar to the conventional dressing group, the VAC therapy was continued until the wounds were healthy and clean and could be closed with meshed grafts or advancement flaps. Although the VAC therapy group was associated with significantly longer hospitalization is was also associated with lower mortality. Although the authors state that their study does not demonstrate that VAC dressings are superior to conventional dressings in terms of length of stay or clinical outcome, they state that "experience has shown that vacuum dressings are clinically effective and successfully used in the management of large wounds". It is important to note that although this study did compare two groups it was not randomized, although the authors do address this point by correctly stating that it would be practically impossible to perform a randomized controlled trial on this group of patients because of the rarity of Fournier's gangrene.

8. Complications

The complications of Fournier's gangrene can include single or multi-organ failure, as well as large scrotal, peri-anal, penile and abdominal wall skin defects. As mentioned previously, Fournier's gangrene may involve the testes, and single or bilateral orchidectomy may need to be performed. The penis may need to be partially or completely amputated in cases of severe gangrene (Schneider et al., 1986). Fournier's gangrene may be the presenting feature of diabetes mellitus, and may be associated with keto-acidosis (Slater et al., 1982). Long-term pain is not uncommon in Fournier's gangrene and 50% of patients can be expected to be free of pain. The sexual function may be impaired by penile deviation or penile torsion as well as loss of sensitivity to the penile skin or pain during erection (Ferreira et al., 2007). Infertility is rare after Fournier's gangrene, but has been reported (Baskin et al., 1990).

9. Conclusion

Fournier's gangrene is a rare necrotising fasciitis of the genitalia originally described in healthy young men. Recent evidence has shown that a cause for the condition can be identified in most patients and today's cohort are unlikely to be healthy young men but elderly patients with co-morbid conditions such as diabetes, immunosuppression or alcoholism. The most common sources of infection are perineal and genital skin infections, although other factors have been implicated in the aetiology of the disease such as pelvic or perineal injury, pelvic interventions and colorectal diseases such as neoplasia or diverticulitis. As outlined above, Fournier's gangrene demonstrates a wide variety of clinical presentations from slow insidious progression of scrotal swelling and pain over weeks to a rapid and fulminant onset within hours. Patients with full-blown Fournier's gangrene usually have pronounced systemic signs such as tachycardia, tachypnoea, fever and possibly altered mental state. Although a wide variety of bacteria have been implicated in the disease (and the disease is frequently polymicrobial) the most common organisms isolated are Staphylococcus aureus, β-haemolytic Streptococcus, Pseudomonas sp., E. coli, Enterococcus and Bacteroides. The spread of infection is along fascial planes and is usually rapid so prompt medical and surgical therapy is mandatory. The mainstay of treatment is early recognition of the disease, prompt resuscitation with intravenous fluids and oxygen therapy, broad-spectrum high dose intravenous antibiotics, and urgent surgical debridement of affected areas. If there is any doubt about the diagnosis of the condition, radiology may be helpful in identifying gas forming organisms or areas of necrosis, and CT has been shown to be particularly helpful in this regard, as well as demonstrating accurately the extent of the disease, and the underlying cause. Due to their separate blood supply the testes are usually spared in Fournier's gangrene and wide areas of skin necrosis may involve debridement of the scrotum, penis, thighs and anterior abdominal wall. Frequently more than one surgical debridement is necessary as a 'second look' at 24-48 hours reveals further areas of necrosis. Once the patient has been stabilised and there is evidence of granulation tissue forming in the debrided areas further treatment can now be instigated. Skin grafting, local and fee flaps have all been used with success in covering areas of debridement after Fournier's gangrene. Recently, VAC (Vaccum Assisted Closure) therapy has been used with promising results in Fournier's gangrene after debridement.

Although early series reported high mortality rates for Fournier's gangrene at around 80% (Stephens et al., 1993) more recent studies have shown an improvement with lower rates of mortality of generally less than 40% (Morpurgo, 2002, Thwaini et al., 2006). Long-term complications of this disease are not uncommon. Pain, sexual dysfunction, incontinence, scarring, and infertility have all been reported.

10. References

Ayan, F., Sunamak, O., Paksoy, S., Polat, S., AS, A., Sakoglu, N., Cetinkale, O. & Sirin, F. 2005. Fournier's gangrene: a retrospective clinical study on forty-one patients. *ANZ journal of surgery*, 75, 1055.

Baskin, L., Carroll, P., Cattolica, E. & Mcaninch, J. 1990. Necrotising soft tissue infections of the perineum and genitalia: Bacteriology, treatment and risk assessment. *British Journal of Urology*, 65, 524-529.

Begley, M., Shawker, T., Robertson, C., Bock, S., Wei, J. & Lotze, M. 1988. Fournier gangrene: diagnosis with scrotal US. *Radiology*, 169, 387.

Campos, J. & Martos, J. 1990. Synchronous caverno-spongious thrombosis and Fournier's gangrene. *Archivos espa√±oles de urolog√a*, 43, 423.

Clayton, M., Fowler JR, J., Sharifi, R. & Pearl, R. 1990. Causes, presentation and survival of fifty-seven patients with necrotizing fasciitis of the male genitalia. *Surgery, gynecology & obstetrics*, 170, 49.

Czymek, R., Schmidt, A., Eckmann, C., Bouchard, R., Wulff, B., Laubert, T., Limmer, S., Bruch, H. P. & Kujath, P. 2009. Fournier's gangrene: vacuum-assisted closure versus conventional dressings. *The American journal of surgery*, 197, 168-176.

Eke, N. 2000. Fourniers gangrene: a review of 1726 cases. *Br J Surg*, 87, 718-728.

Elliott, D., Kufera, J. A. & Myers, R. A. M. 2000. The microbiology of necrotizing soft tissue infections. *The American journal of surgery*, 179, 361-366.

Ersay, A., Yilmaz, G., Akgun, Y. & Celik, Y. 2007. Factors affecting mortality of Fournierís gangrene: review of 70 patients. *ANZ journal of surgery*, 77, 43-48.

Ferreira, P. C., Reis, J. C., Amarante, J. M., Silva, A. C., Pinho, C. J., Oliveira, I. C. & Da Silva, P. N. 2007. Fournier's gangrene: a review of 43 reconstructive cases. *Plastic and reconstructive surgery*, 119, 175.

Fournier, J. 1883. Gangrene foudroyante de la verge. *Semaine Med*, 3, 345.

Gupta, A., Dalela, D., Sankhwar, S., Goel, M., Kumar, S., Goel, A. & Singh, V. 2007. Bilateral testicular gangrene: does it occur in Fournier's gangrene? *Int Urol Nephrol*, 39, 913-915.

Hejase, M. J., Simonin, J. E., Bihrle, R. & Coogan, C. L. 1996. Genital Fournier's gangrene: experience with 38 patients. *Urology*, 47, 734-739.

Korhonen, K., Hirn, M. & Niinikoski, J. 1998. Hyperbaric oxygen in the treatment of Fournier's gangrene. *European Journal of Surgery*, 164, 251-255.

Korkut, M., Á^Z, G., Dayangaá, M., Akg¸N, E., Yeniay, L., Erdo AN & «AL 2003. Outcome analysis in patients with Fournierís gangrene. *Diseases of the Colon & Rectum*, 46, 649-652.

Kuo, C., Wang, W., Lee, C., Liu, C. & Tseng, H. 2007. Fournier's gangrene: ten-year experience in a medical center in northern Taiwan. *J Microbiol Immunol Infect,* 40, 500-506.

Laor, E., Palmer, L. S., Tolia, B. M., Reid, R. E. & Winter, H. I. 1995. Outcome prediction in patients with Fournier's gangrene. *The Journal of urology,* 154, 89-92.

Laucks II, S. 1994. Fournier's gangrene. *The Surgical clinics of North America,* 74, 1339.

Levenson, R. B., Singh, A. K. & Novelline, R. A. 2008. Fournier gangrene: role of imaging.

Lowthian, J. T. & Gillard JR, L. J. 1980. Postpartum necrotizing fasciitis. *Obstetrics & Gynecology,* 56, 661.

Morpurgo, E. 2002. Galandiuk S. Fournierís gangrene. *Surg Clin North Am,* 82, 1213-24.

Omotoso, A. 1990. Aderibigbe A. Fournierís gangrene complicated by tetanus: case report. *Orient J Med,* 2, 207-8.

Ozden Yeniyol, C., Suelozgen, T., Arslan, M. & Riza Ayder, A. 2004. Fournier's gangrene: experience with 25 patients and use of Fournier's gangrene severity index score. *Urology,* 64, 218-222.

Randall, A. 1920. Idiopathic gangrene of the scrotum. *J Urol,* 4, 219.

Russell, R. C. G., Williams, N. S. & Bulstrode, C. J. K. 2000. *Bailey & Love's short practice of surgery,* Arnold.

Rye, B., Seidelin, C. & Dueholm, S. 1987. Perineal progressive myonecrosis following Thiersch's operation for rectal prolapse. *Ann Chir Gynaecol,* 76, 136-137.

Safioleas, M., Stamatakos, M., Mouzopoulos, G., Diab, A., Kontzoglou, K. & Papachristodoulou, A. 2006. Fournierís gangrene: exists and it is still lethal. *International urology and nephrology,* 38, 653-657.

Saijo, S., Kuramoto, Y., Yoshinari, M. & TAGAMI, H. 1990. Extremely extended Fournier's gangrene. *Dermatologica,* 181, 228.

Schneider, P. R., Russell, R. C. & Zook, E. G. 1986. Fournier's gangrene of the penis: a report of two cases. *Annals of plastic surgery,* 17, 87.

Slater, D., Smith, G. & Mundy, K. 1982. Diabetes mellitus with ketoacidosis presenting as Fournier's gangrene. *Journal of the Royal Society of Medicine,* 75, 530.

Stephens, B., Lathrop, J., Rice, W. & Gruenberg, J. 1993. Fournier's gangrene: historic (1764-1978) versus contemporary (1979-1988) differences in etiology and clinical importance. *The American surgeon,* 59, 149-154.

Thomas, J. 1956. Fournier's gangrene of the penis and the scrotum. *The Journal of urology,* 75, 719.

Thwaini, A., Khan, A., Malik, A., Cherian, J., Barua, J., Shergill, I. & Mammen, K. 2006. Fournierís gangrene and its emergency management. *Postgraduate medical journal,* 82, 516.

Wolach, M., Macdermott, J., Stone, A. & White, R. 1989. Treatment and complications of Fournier's gangrene. *British Journal of Urology,* 64, 310-314.

Wong, C. H., Khin, L. W., Heng, K. S., Tan, K. C. & Low, C. O. 2004. The LRINEC (Laboratory Risk Indicator for Necrotizing Fasciitis) score: A tool for distinguishing necrotizing fasciitis from other soft tissue infections*. *Critical care medicine,* 32, 1535.

Woodside, J. R. 1980. Necrotizing fasciitis after neonatal circumcision. *Am J Dis Child,* 134, 301-2.

Wysoki, M. G., Santora, T. A., Shah, R. M. & Friedman, A. C. 1997. Necrotizing fasciitis: CT characteristics. *Radiology*, 203, 859.

3

Perineal Gangrene: Clinical and Therapeutic Features and Pronostic Analysis of 35 Cases

Slim Jarboui, Ayoub Zoghlami and Dorsaf Othmani
University of medicine - Tunis
Tunisia

1. Introduction

Perineal gangrene is a cellulo-fasciitis secondary to a polymicrobial infection whose evolving is rapidly changing and unpredictable. Its prognosis is poor in spite of an appropriate therapeutic management. We have analyzed retrospectively 35 consecutive cases of perineal gangrene treated in the "A" surgical department of Charles Nicolle hospital (Tunisia). Our aim was to describe the clinical and therapeutic features and to analyze the prognostic factors that may influence the postoperative course.

2. Methods

Our retrospective study analysed 35 consecutive cases of perineal gangrene treated in the "A" surgical department of Charles Nicolle hospital (Tunisia) between 1997 and 2004. All the cases of perineal gangrene were included whatever the gateway: proctologic, urogenital, post-traumatic or postoperative. Gangrene that did not reach the perineum and perianal suppuration without cellulitis nor myonecrosis mentioned on the operative report were excluded. For each patient we studied age, sex, medical history, risk factors, etiology, diagnosis delay, topography, extent of lesions, clinical severity signs, results of laboratory workup and morphological examination. The therapeutic armamentarium consisted of intensive care including the correction of hypovolemia and electrolyte disorders, antibiotic therapy against anaerobic bacteria, gram-negative bacilli and gram-positive cocci, and surgical treatment consisting of iterative excisions, drainage, dressing change in the operating room and stomas if necessary.

The simplified severity index in its second version (SSI II) and the Fournier gangrene severity index score (FGSIS) were calculated from clinical and biological parameters in order to assess the severity of the initial clinical syndrome and to include these scores in a prognostic analysis. A univariate analysis using SPSS 11.5 was performed to search for prognostic factors that could influence mortality. Then we tried, through a multivariate analysis to identify independent risk factors with a significance level of 0.05.

3. Results

Between 1997 and 2004, 35 patients with perineal gangrene were supported in the "A" surgical department of Charles Nicolle hospital. The average age was 50.3 (± 14.1), there were 25 men and 10 women. 23 patients had diabetes, 10 had hypertension. Regarding the etiology, 18 (51.4%) had perianal suppurations, 9 (25.7%) had abscesses of the buttock, and 5 had a urogenital infection. Time before diagnosis ranged from 3 to 30 days with an average of 12.71 (± 8.37) days. Among the initial symptoms, perineal pain was found in 30 patients (85.7%), pyrexia was found in 31 patients (88.6%). One patient had initial shock (case n°4). Bacterial gas production was revealed by subcutaneous crackling found in 3 patients (8.6%) (Cases n°2, 4 and 22), or by signs in the radiography found in one case (case n°2). Leukocytosis (white blood cell count >10 000/mm^3) was found in 29 patients (82.9%). The anatomic lesions consisted in cellulitis and myonecrosis in 34.2% cases. The extent of cellulitis and myonecrosis are represented in figures 1 and 2. All the patients had an almost-standardized treatment protocol consisting in 3 main measures: intensive care, antibiotic therapy and surgery. Intensive care comprised volume expansion, oxygen therapy and correction of metabolic and electrolytic disorders. Transurethral catheterization was performed in 7 patients while 3 patients had suprapubic catheterization. Antibiotic therapy was introduced since the admission. It was a tentative therapy covering anaerobic bacteria, gram-negative bacilli and gram-positive-cocci. The combination penicillin-gentamicin-metronidazole was prescribed in 88.5% cases. Ofloxacin was used when patients were allergic to beta-lactam antibiotics. None of our patients had hyperbaric oxygen therapy. Surgery was performed under general anaesthesia and comprised wide cutaneous, subcutaneous and muscle excisions up to healthy limits. Washing with hydrogen peroxide was always used. Wounds were left widely opened and corrugated drainage sets were used in the subcutaneous and muscle detachments. 30 patients (85.7% cases) had iterative excisions under general anaesthesia. The number of excisions ranged from 1 to 11 with an average of 3.2 ±2.9. 2 patients had lateral colosigmoidostomy because of a huge circumferential decay of the anal canal and the rectum (cases n°3 and 16). Postoperative mortality affected 6 patients (17.1%). The average age of deceased patients was 54. Characteristics of these patients are summarized in table I. Deaths were secondary to septic shock in 4 patients. Decompensation of a previous disease led to death in 2 cases. Death occurred between day 1 and day 39 after surgery. Length of stay ranged from 2 to 64 days with an average of 15.31 days ±13.29.

The postoperative course was complicated in 9 patients (25.7%) secondary to decompensation of previous diseases (table I). Restoration of continuity was performed in 2 patients (cases n°3 and 16) within respectively 9 and 13 months with no additional morbidity. One case of anal incontinence was noted as a postoperative sequela (case n°8). No urogenital sequelae were observed. The univariate analysis (table II) showed that mortality was significantly influenced by the spread of cellulitis, the presence of myonecrosis, the occurrence of septic shock, the postoperative need for mechanical ventilation and severity scores (SSI II and FGSIS). The multivariate study did not identify any independent factor of mortality.

4. Discussion

Perineal gangrene is a rare and serious complaint that poses a nosological problem leading to varied terminology: Meleney syndrome, synergistic necrotizing cellulitis, necrotizing fasciitis, clostridial gas gangrene and Fournier's disease [1,2]. It's defined as a necrotizing

Case	Age	Sex	Etiology	Diagnostic delay (days)	SSI II	FGSIS	Number of iterative excisions	Postoperative course
1	63	F	Anal suppuration	10	28	4	2	decompensation
2	29	M	Anal suppuration	9	19	5	10	uneventful
3	65	F	Bartholinitis	21	45	17	5	decease
4	43	M	Anal suppuration	7	59	13	0	decease
5	60	M	Abscess of buttock	30	20	1	4	uneventful
6	30	M	Scrotal infection	15	11	3	5	uneventful
7	67	M	Anal suppuration	10	38	9	1	decease
8	54	M	Anal suppuration	17	21	4	1	uneventful
9	49	M	Anal suppuration	23	15	3	0	decompensation
10	36	M	Abscess of buttock	7	11	4	4	uneventful
11	66	M	Anal suppuration	10	20	1	7	decompensation
12	45	F	Anal suppuration	15	18	4	1	uneventful
13	48	F	Inguinal lymphadenitis	30	38	13	2	decease
14	51	M	Bedsores	30	33	7	0	decease
15	57	M	Abscess of buttock	7	15	4	2	uneventful
16	22	M	Post-trauma	13	15	9	11	uneventful
17	77	M	Anal suppuration	7	44	0	0	uneventful
18	52	F	Bartholinitis	7	21	2	2	decompensation

Case	Age	Sex	Etiology	Diagnostic delay (days)	SSI II	FGSIS	Number of iterative excisions	Postoperative course
19	61	M	Anal suppuration	10	26	3	1	uneventful
20	47	M	Anal suppuration	7	18	3	2	decompensation
21	76	M	Abscess of buttock	21	4	0	2	uneventful
22	43	M	Anal suppuration	3	18	2	2	decompensation
23	63	M	Anal suppuration	7	20	1	1	uneventful
24	29	F	Abscess of buttock	30	33	7	3	uneventful
25	57	F	Bartholinitis	3	18	7	2	decompensation
26	25	F	Anal suppuration	7	14	5	3	uneventful
27	50	M	Anal suppuration	24	15	1	1	uneventful
28	58	F	Anal suppuration	15	21	5	1	uneventful
29	26	M	Anal suppuration	6	10	11	1	uneventful
30	55	M	Abscess of buttock	6	20	5	6	uneventful
31	41	M	Abscess of buttock	6	16	0	0	uneventful
32	53	M	Abscess of buttock	7	18	4	1	decompensation
33	61	F	Anal suppuration	15	26	5	1	uneventful
34	52	M	Scrotal infection	5	15	0	1	uneventful
35	50	M	Abscess of buttock	5	18	4	10	decease

SSI II: simplified severity index in its second version; FGSIS: Fournier gangrene severity score index

Table 1. Characteristics of studied cases

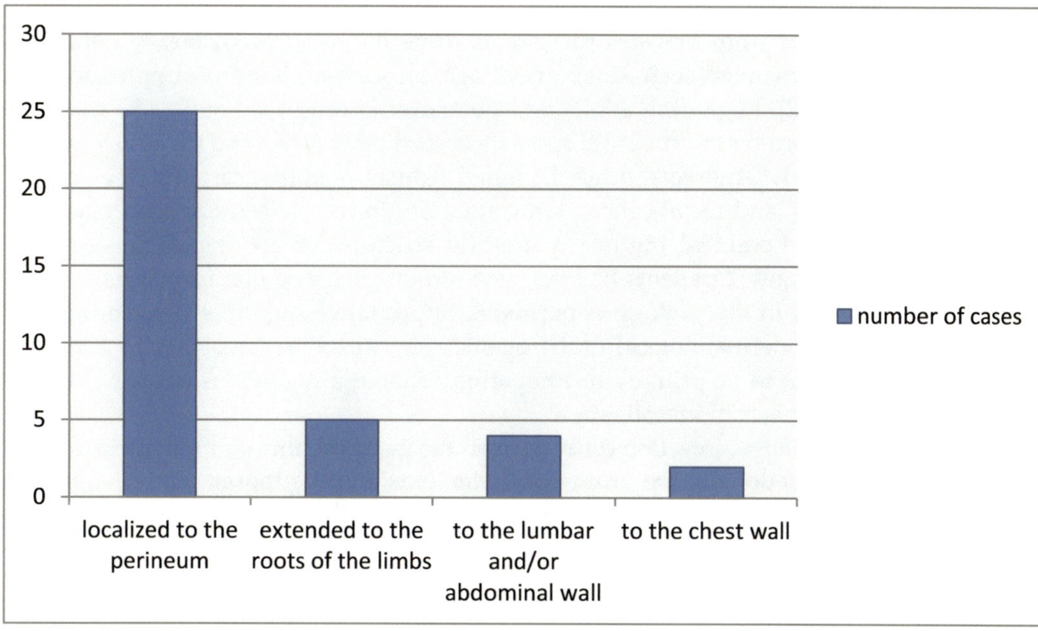

Fig. 1. Extent of cellulitis

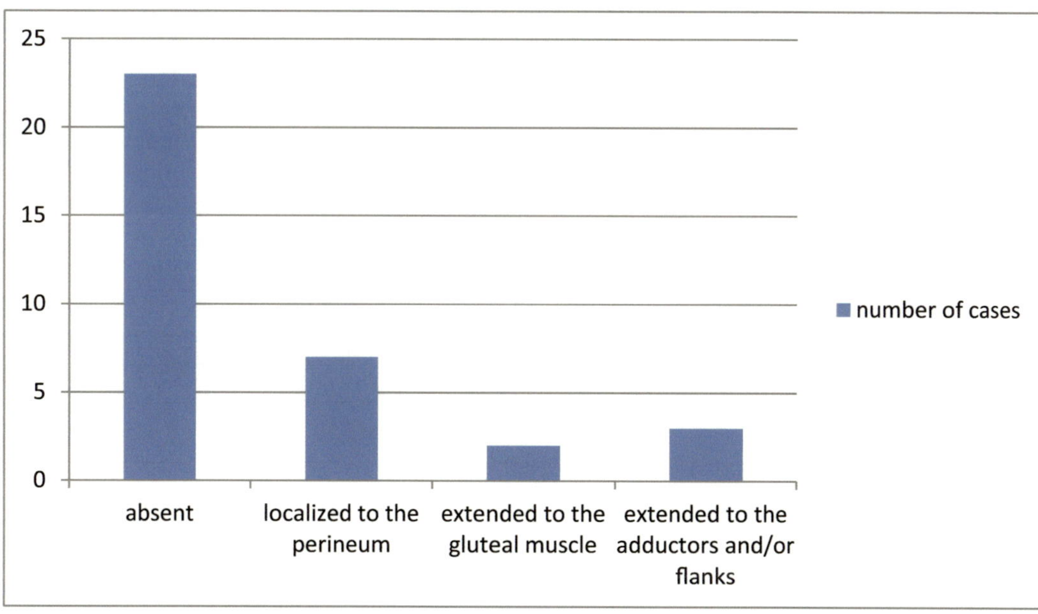

Fig. 2. Extent of myonecrosis

cellulo-fasciitis of perineum and external genitalia. This disease can occur at any age but predominates between 40 and 50. In our series, the average age was 50.3 with predominance in males (71.4%). Apart from diabetes that seems to be the main predisposing condition, other risk factors are involved such as advanced age, alcoholism, immunosuppression and neoplastic diseases [1,2]. Regarding etiologies, the anorectal origin seemed to be the more frequent one: 37% according to Brunet [2] and 42% according to Al Mejjad [3]. This rate rises up to 62.8% in our study. Anorectal origin included fistulas, anal fissures, abscesses of anal margin, sexual injuries, and rectal cancer. Urogenital origin comes in the second place and may consist in a pelvi-perineal trauma, a urethral stricture, or an epididymo-testicular abscess. In our series, only 2 patients had perineal scrotal gangrene because, in most cases, patients are supported in the urology department. Suppurative digestive diseases such as sigmoid diverticulitis, dermatological or iatrogenic origin may be involved. In 5 to 35% cases, gangrene seemed to be primary or idiopathic, without any obvious etiology because of delayed diagnosis or lack of investigation.

Regarding pathophysiology, infection diffuses from the gateway, through the fascia and the cellular spaces to the abdomen, the groin areas, the loins and the thorax. Bacterial growth leads to microvasculitis which leads to healing of the capillary flow causing microthrombosis and necrosis. The extensive cellulo-fasciitis is due to two main facts. On the one hand, the loose texture of fatty tissues facilitates the spread of infection; on the other hand, the perineum is a real anatomical crossroads which communicates with the ischiorectal fossa, the gluteal region, the iliac fossa, the lumbar wall and the anterior abdominal wall. Regarding bacteriology, perineal gangrene is in most cases secondary to a polymicrobial infection involving anaerobic bacteria, gram-negative bacilli and gram-positive cocci. It's considered as a typical model of bacterial synergy [1, 2]. Indeed, aerobic bacteria consume oxygen and create an environment conducive to the growth of anaerobic bacteria. The most frequently isolated germs are: Escherichia coli, Bacteroides fragilis, streptococcus, staphylococcus, Pseudomonas and Clostridium. Sometimes, fungi are involved [4]. These pathogenic organisms are not always isolated. Clinically, the diagnosis is often delayed many days or even weeks in most series including ours (about 13 days on average). It's actually a factor correlated to a poorer prognosis and to a locally advanced disease with erythema, edema, cellulitis, myonecrosis, and general signs of infection such as chills, pyrexia and even septic shock. Crackling is pathognomonic but not mandatory. It was found in 3 patients in our series, 13/31 in El Mejjad's [3]. Imaging may be useful but should not delay the therapeutic management. Radiography can show aeric clarities in the subcutaneous tissues. Ultrasonography shows infiltrated tissues with hyper echoic areas [5, 6]. Computed tomography precises the starting point of the gangrene and assesses its extent in order to adapt surgery [1, 3]. In our series, only one patient had a radiography that showed aeric clarities in the wall. The other patients were examined at an advanced stage thus all additional tests would have been superfluous. Perineal gangrene is a therapeutic emergency. It necessitates a fast and sometimes highly aggressive management. This management comprises [1, 2, 7, 8] intensive care. Antibiotic therapy is systematically introduced and it's based on a broad-spectrum combination against gram-negative, gram-positive and anaerobic germs. It's secondarily adapted to the antibiogram. The more prescribed combination is beta lactam-aminoglycoside-metronidazole (88% in our study). Surgery consists of debridement and excision of damaged tissues up to healthy margins. We advocate, as for most authors, a highly aggressive surgical debridement since the very first operation, even at the expense of a wide tissue sacrifice. Some authors recommend a more conservative management [9-11]. According to Brunet [2, 8], this open surgery should not leave any focus of infection which could act as a starting point to septic outbreaks. He recommends also a systematic exploration of the ischiorectal fossa. Colostomy is mandatory for some authors [2, 8], optional for others. It's indicated for severe perineal gangrene or when the gateway is proctologic [3, 9]. Colostomy avoids fecal contamination of the wound and facilitates local care and healing. It has two requirements: the colonic segment excluded should be as short as possible, and avoid externalizing the stoma in an area reached by gangrene. In our series, colostomy was performed twice. Despite its benefits described above, it didn't seem to influence the post-operative course for our patients. For Brunet's team, colostomy is systematically performed on the right transverse colon. No additional morbidity is reported when continuity is restored. It should be performed only once the wound heals and after making sure of the continence of the anal sphincter. Iterative excisions in the operating room are quite often necessary, in addition to the initial excision. Transurethral or suprapubic catheterization may be necessary when the gateway is urological but can expose to the diffusion of infection to the bladder and to the upper urinary tract [1]. In our series, 3 patients had suprapubic catheterization and 6 had transurethral catheterization. In the perineal gangrene, testicles and erectile bodies are generally spared. Necrosis of the testicles imposes an orchiectomy and a laparotomy in search of the cause of thrombosis of spermatic vessels [9]. Some clinical studies have shown that Vacuum dressing is particularly effective in the management of large wounds. This was associated with longer hospitalization and lower mortality [12].

Once the systemic septic risk controlled and the wound healed, procedures of secondary covering can be performed using cutaneous, fasciocutaneous and musculocutaneous flaps or approximation suture [1, 13]. Regarding prognosis, perineal gangrene is a serious disease whose mortality ranges from 20 to 50%. This mortality is worsened by delayed therapeutic management, previous debilitating diseases and septic shock. Prognostic factors do vary from a series to another. In ours, the univariate analysis identified many factors which could influence mortality such as the extent of cellulitis, the presence of myonecrosis, the occurrence of a septic shock, the postoperative need for mechanical ventilation and severity scores (SSI II and FGSIS). Diagnosis delay did not seem to be a prognostic factor: 11.8 days for survivors versus 17.2 days for deceased (p=0.15). In other series, advanced age [9], diagnostic and therapeutic delay [2, 3], the extent of myonecrosis [2], FGSIS [10, 11] and SSI II [2], positive culture for streptococcus [1] have been identified as factors correlated to a poor prognosis.

5. Conclusion

Perineal gangrene is an uncommon but life threatening condition with high associated mortality and morbidity. Early diagnosis and aggressive surgical debridement are the main treatment.

6. References

[1] Cadot P, Rouquette I, Szym P, André JL. Les cellulites graves, ou gangrène de Fournier du périnée. J Chir 2003;140:22-32.

[2] Brunet C, Consentino B, Barthelemy A, Huart L. Gangrènes périnéales : nouvelles approches bactériologiques. Résultats du traitement médicochirurgical (81 cas). Ann Chir 2000;125:420-7.
[3] El Mejjad A, Belmahi A, Choukri A, Kafih M. La gangrène périnéo-scrotale : à propos de 31 cas. Ann Urol 2002;36:277-85.
[4] Kazuyoshi J, Masaki N, Takashi K. Fournier's gangrene caused by Candida species as the primary organism. Urology 2000; 56:153.
[5] Özhan Oktar S, Yücel C, Tokgöz Ercan N, Çapkan D, Özdemir H. Fournier's gangrene: US and MR imaging findings. Eur J Radiol 2004; 50:81-7.
[6] Morrison D, Blaivas M, Lyon M. Emergency diagnosis of Fournier's gangrene with bedside ultrasound. Am J Emerg Med 2005; 23:544-7.
[7] Riseman JA. Hyperbaric oxygen therapy for necrotizing fasciitis reduces mortality and the need for debridements. Surgery 1990;154:847-50.
[8] Brunet C, Dlpero JR, Guerinel G, Geisser A, Barthélémy A, Sainty JM et al. Gangrènes du périnée. Plaidoyer pour une conduite thérapeutique standardisé à propos de 50 observations. Chirurgie 1992;118: 607-14.
[9] Tazi K, Karmouni T, El Fassi J, El khader K. Gangrène périnéoscrotale : à propos de 51 cas. Aspects diagnostiques et thérapeutiques. Ann Urol 2001;35:229-33.
[10] Cem Ozden Y, Tufan S, Murat A. Fournier's gangrene: experience with 25 patients and use of Fournier's Gangrene Severity Index Score. Urology 2004; 64:218-22.
[11] Chawla SN, Gallop C, Mydlo JH. Fournier's gangrene: An analysis of repeated surgical debridement. Eur Urol 2003;43: 572-5.
[12] Czymek R, Schmidt A, Eckmann C, Boucher R, Wulff B, Laubert T? and All. Fournier's Gangrene: Vacuum-Assisted Closure versus Conventional Dressing. The American Jornal of Surgery 2009; 197:168-176.
[13] Verna G, Fava F, Baglioni E, Cannatà M, Devalle L, Fraccalvieri M. La gangrène de Fournier : remarques sur deux cas cliniques. Ann Chir Plast Esthet 2003;49: 37-42.

4

Fournier's Gangrene

Ndubuisi Eke and John E. Raphael
Urology Unit, Department of Surgery, University of Port Harcourt Teaching Hospital, Port Harcourt, Nigeria

1. Introduction

Fournier's gangrene (FG) is an acute, rapidly progressive and potentially fatal, infective necrotizing fasciitis affecting the external genitalia, perineal or perianal regions[1]. The definition of FG changed more often than the treatment over the years. Professor Jean-Alfred Fournier (1832-1914), first defined FG as an 'acute idiopathic gangrene of the scrotum in the young male[2]. The frequent isolation of causative organisms led to the first modification. Observation that the elderly with certain co-morbidities are more often affected along with reports in women went a long way in modifying the description of FG[3].

FG is a disease of antiquity. King Herod of Judea was suspected to have suffered from genital gangrene in association with diabetes mellitus [4]. Over the decades, FG has proved to be an enigma to the physician and an embarrassment to the patient. In 1764, Baurienne originally described an idiopathic, rapidly progressive soft-tissue necrotizing process that led to gangrene of the male genitalia. However, Jean-Alfred Fournier, a Parisian venereologist, is more commonly associated with this disease, which bears his name. In one of Fournier's clinical lectures in 1883, he presented a case of perineal gangrene in an otherwise healthy young man[5]. Since Fournier's description, subsequent experience has shown that, in most cases, Fournier gangrene has an identifiable cause and that it frequently manifests more indolently. Trauma to the genitalia continues to be a frequently recognized vector for the introduction of bacteria that initiate the infectious process[5]. The disease carries a significant mortality. The mortality from FG has shown no correlation with advancement in medical services. An unpublished report indicates a paradoxically higher mortality rate in developed countries compared to developing ones.

2. Epidemiology

Fournier's gangrene is relatively uncommon. The true incidence of the disease is unknown. However, the incidence appears to be rising. In a retrospective study of cases reported in the English literature from 1950-1999, 1726 cases were documented[6]. A continuing study on Fournier's gangrene, yet to be published, revealed 1571 cases from 2000 to 2007. This rise may partly be attributed to the exploitation of the internet to disseminate information[7]. Most reported cases occur in patients aged 30-60 years. A literature review found only 56 paediatric cases, with 66% of those in infants younger than 3 months.

Earlier reports excluded women, probably because Fournier's original report, from which the disease got its eponym, excluded women and children. The male-to-female ratio is approximately 10:1. Lower incidence in females may not be unrelated to better drainage of the perineal region through vaginal secretions. Male homosexuals may be at higher risk, especially to drug resistant strains[8].

3. Relevant anatomy

The corpora, urethra, testes, and cord structures are usually not involved in Fournier's gangrene, while the superficial and deep fascia and the skin are destroyed. The complex anatomy of the male external genitalia influences the initiation and progression of Fournier's gangrene. This infectious process involves the superficial and deep fascial planes of the genitalia. As the microorganisms responsible for the infection multiply, infection spreads along the anatomical fascial planes, often sparing the deep muscular structures and, to variable degrees, the overlying skin. The knowledge of the peculiar anatomy of the male lower urinary tract and external genitalia is critical for the clinician treating a man with Fournier's gangrene.

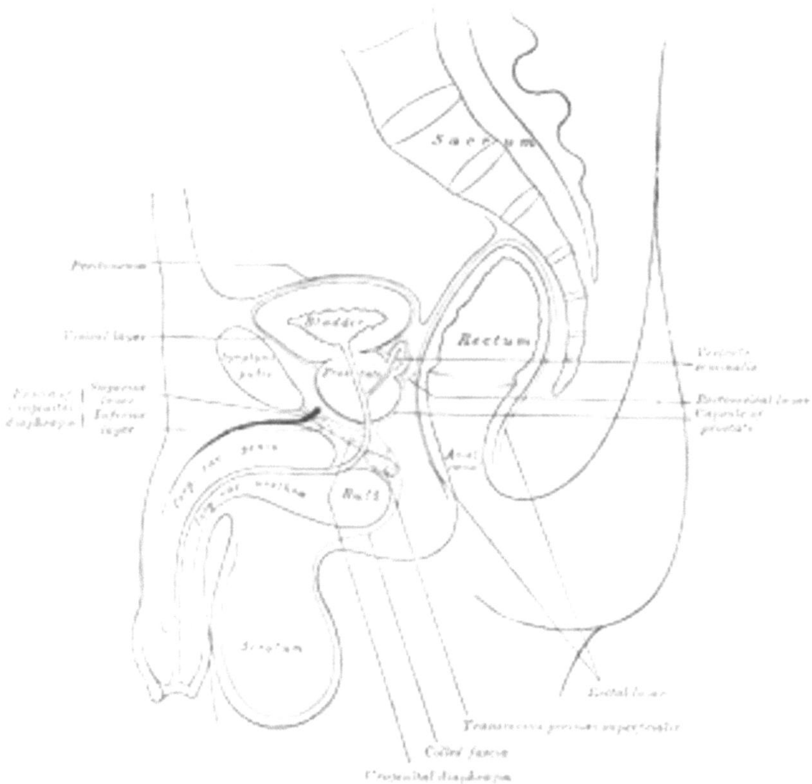

Fig. 1. Fascial arrangement of the scrotum and perineum[9]

Colles' fascia completely envelops the scrotum and penis, continuiting cephalad to the level of the clavicles. In the inguinal region, this fascial layer is known as Scarpa's fascia. Understanding the tendency of necrotizing fasciitis to spread along fascial planes and the fascial anatomy, one can see how a process that initiates in the perineum can spread to the abdominal wall, the flank, and even the chest wall.

4. Skin and superficial fascia

Because Fournier's gangrene is predominantly an infectious process of the superficial and deep fascial planes, appreciating the anatomic relationship of the skin and subcutaneous structures of the perineum and abdominal wall is vital.

The skin cephalad to the inguinal ligament is backed by Camper's fascia, which is a layer of fat-containing tissue of varying thickness and the superficial vessels to the skin that run through it. Scarpa's fascia forms another distinct layer deep to Camper fascia. In the perineum, Scarpa's fascia blends into Colles' fascia (superficial perineal fascia), and continuous with Dartos fascia of the penis and scrotum.

Several important anatomic relationships should be considered. A potential space between the Scarpa's fascia and the deep fascia of the anterior wall (external abdominal oblique) allows for the extension of a perineal infection into the anterior abdominal wall. Superiorly, Scarpa's and Camper's fasciae coalesce and attach to the clavicles, ultimately limiting the cephalad extension of an infection that may have originated in the perineum. Colles's fascia is attached to the pubic arch and the base of the perineal membrane, and it is continuous with the superficial Dartos fascia of the scrotal wall. The perineal membrane is also known as the inferior fascia of the urogenital diaphragm and, together with Colles' fascia, defines the superficial perineal space.

This space contains the membranous urethra, bulbar urethra, and bulbourethral glands. In addition, this space is adjacent to the anterior anal wall and ischiorectal fossae. Infectious disease of the male urethra, bulbourethral glands, perineal structures, or rectum can drain into the superficial perineal space and can extend into the scrotum or into the anterior abdominal wall up to the level of the clavicles.

5. Blood supply

Branches from the inferior epigastric and deep circumflex iliac arteries supply the lower aspect of the anterior abdominal wall. Branches of the external and internal pudendal arteries supply the scrotal wall. With the exception of the internal pudendal artery, each of these vessels travels within Camper's fascia and can therefore become thrombosed in the pathogenesis of Fournier gangrene.

In the male, the testis receives its blood supply primarily from the testicular artery, a branch of the abdominal aorta. This explains the sparing of the testis in Fournier's gangrene.

Thrombosis jeopardizes the viability of the skin of the scrotum and perineum. Often, the posterior aspect of the scrotal wall supplied by the internal pudendal artery remains viable and can be used in the reconstruction following resolution of the infection.

6. Penis and scrotum

The contents of the scrotum, namely the testes, epididymides and cord structures, are invested by several fascial layers distinct from the Dartos fascia of the scrotal wall.

The most superficial layer of the testis and cord is the external spermatic fascia, which is continuous with the external oblique aponeurosis of the superficial inguinal ring . The next deeper layer is the internal spermatic fascia, which is continuous with the transversalis fascia. The Buck fascia covers the erectile bodies of the penis, the corpora cavernosa, and the anterior urethra. The Buck fascia fuses to the dense tunica albuginea of the corpora cavernosa, deep in the pelvis. These fascial layers do not become involved with an infection of the superficial perineal space and can limit the depth of tissue destruction in a necrotizing infection of the genitalia.

7. Aetiology

Although originally described as idiopathic gangrene of the genitalia, Fournier gangrene has an identifiable cause in approximately 95% of cases. The necrotizing process commonly originates from an infection in the anorectum, urogenital tract, or skin of the genitalia [10]. Trauma, recent surgery, and the presence of foreign bodies may also lead to the disease. Perianal, perirectal and ischiorectal abscesses, anal fissures; colonic perforations, urethral strictures with urinary extravasations; epididymoorchitis or hidradenitis may lead to the disease. Urethral instrumentation, prosthetic penile implants, superficial soft-tissue injuries, intramuscular injections, genital piercings, steroid enemas (used for the treatment of radiation proctitis), blunt thoracic trauma, and penile self-injection with cocaine have been reported in the literature as causative factors.

In women, septic abortions, vulva or Bartholin gland abscesses, hysterectomy, and episiotomy are documented sources of sepsis. In men, anal intercourse may increase risk of perineal infection, either from blunt trauma to the area or by spread of rectally carried microbes.

In children, strangulated inguinal hernia, circumcision, omphalitis, insect bites, trauma, urethral instrumentation, peri-rectal abscesses, systemic infections, and burns have led to the disease.

Poor perineal hygiene or the presence of chronically indwelling catheters, such as in paraplegic patients, poses an increased risk.

Wound cultures from patients with Fournier gangrene reveal that it is a polymicrobial infection with an average of four isolates per case. *Escherichia coli* is the predominant aerobe, and *Bacteroides* species the predominant anaerobe. Other common microflora includes *Proteus, Staphylococcus, Enterococcus,* aerobic and anaerobic *Streptococcus, Pseudomonas, Klebsiella,* and *Clostridium.* Incidence of methicillin-resistant *Staphylococcus aureus* (MRSA) may be increasing [7].

Any condition that leads to depressed cellular immunity may predispose a patient to the development of Fournier gangrene. Examples include the following: diabetes mellitus (present in as many as 60% of cases), alcoholism, extremes of age, malignancy, chronic steroid use, cytotoxic drugs, lymphoproliferative diseases, malnutrition and HIV infection.

8. Pathophysiology

The following are pathognomonic findings of Fournier gangrene upon pathologic evaluation of the involved tissue:

Necrosis of the superficial and deep fascial planes,

Fibrinoid coagulation of the nutrient arterioles,

Polymorphonuclear cell infiltration and

Microorganisms identified within the involved tissues

In necrotizing fasciitis as opposed to cellulitis, the location of the inflammation involves the subcutaneous fat, fascia, and muscle in addition to the dermis. A photomicrograph may show the presence of ulcerated epidermis and the presence of thrombosed blood vessel

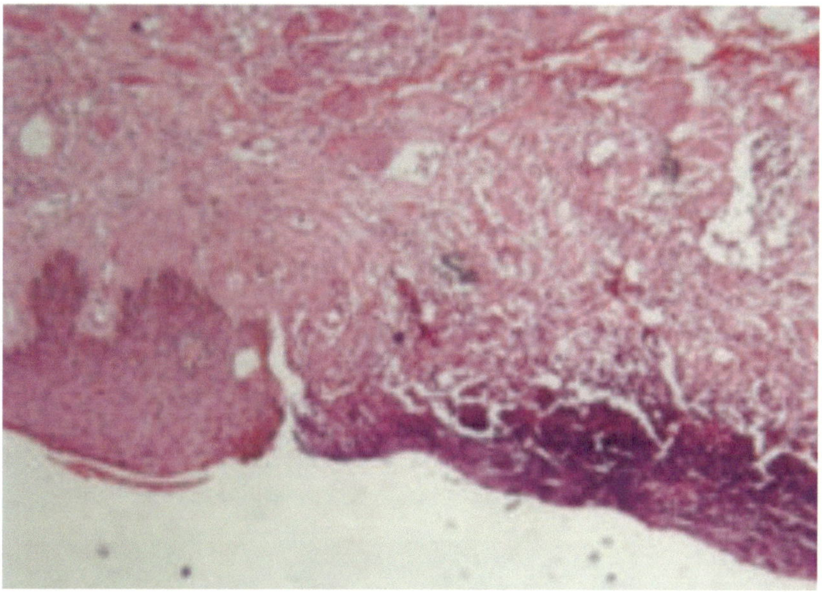

Fig. 2. Ulcerated epidermis and dermis with thrombosed blood vessel and bacterial colonies

Infection represents an imbalance between host immunity and the virulence of the causative microorganisms. The aetiologic factors allow the portal of entry of the microorganism into the perineum. The compromised immunity provides a favourable environment to initiate the infection, and the virulence of the microorganism promotes the rapid spread of the disease. Microorganism virulence results from the production of toxins or enzymes that create an environment conducive to rapid microbial multiplication [11]. In a 1924 series of Chinese men with necrotizing infections, Meleney reported that streptococcal species were the predominant organisms recovered from cultures [12]. Meleney attributed the FG to this sole genus. Subsequent clinical series however stress the polymicrobial nature of most cases of necrotizing infection including Fournier's gangrene [13,14].

Presently, recovering only streptococcal spp is unusual [15]. Rather, streptococcal organisms are culture along with as many as five other organisms. The commonest causative organisms are Streptococcus spp, Staphylococcus spp., Genera of Enterobacteriaceae family, anaerobic organisms and fungi.

Most authorities believe the polymicrobial nature of Fournier gangrene is necessary to create the synergy of enzyme production that promotes rapid multiplication and spread of the infection [11]. For example, one microorganism might produce the enzymes necessary to cause coagulation of the nutrient vessels. Thrombosis of these nutrient vessels reduces local blood supply. Thus, tissue oxygen tension falls. The resultant tissue hypoxia allows growth of facultative anaerobes and microaerophilic organisms. These latter microorganisms, in turn, may produce enzymes (e.g., lecithinase, collagenase), which lead to digestion of fascial barriers, thus fueling the rapid extension of the infection.

The fascial necrosis and digestion are hallmarks of FG. Knowledge of this provides the surgeon with a clinical marker of the extent of tissue affectation. Severe or fulminant Fournier's gangrene can spread from the fascial envelopment of the genitalia throughout the perineum, along the trunk, occasionally, into the thighs and very rarely, to the chest.

9. Clinical presentation

A thorough review of systems, including history of diabetes, alcohol abuse, cancer, colorectal or urogenital disease or surgery, steroid use, sexual history, and HIV status is important. Fournier's gangrene usually begins with an insidious onset of pruritus and discomfort of the external genitalia. Early in the course of the disease, pain may be out of proportion to physical findings. Swelling and erythema of the region follow pain, and a patient may complain of systemic symptoms such as fever or chills. As gangrene develops, pain may subside as nerve tissue becomes necrotic.

Skin overlying the affected region may be normal, erythematous, edematous, cyanotic, bronzed, indurated, blistered, and/or frankly gangrenous. Skin appearance often underestimates the degree of underlying disease. A faeculent odor may be present secondary to infection with anaerobic bacteria. Crepitus may be present, but its absence does not exclude the presence of Clostridium species or other gas-producing organisms. Systemic symptoms (e.g. fever, tachycardia, and hypotension) may be present. A thorough genital and perianal examination is required to detect potential portal of entry.

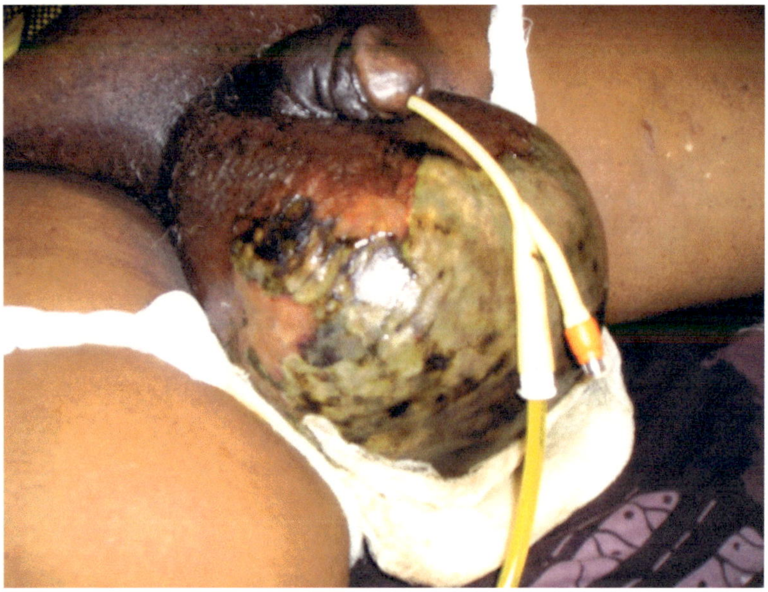

Fig. 3. Fournier's gangrene of the scrotum

10. Investigations

The diagnosis of Fournier's gangrene is clinical and includes the history and physical examination findings, especially the anatomical involvement in the external genitalia and perineum. Urinalysis and blood sugar measurements give evidence of metabolic derangements such as diabetes mellitus. Considering that FG is a urological emergency, treatment should not be delayed for these investigative tools. Other investigations are essential to identify co-morbid factors as well as causative factors. Appropriate bacteriological evaluation of pus from the gangrene, full blood count, renal and hepatic function studies are essential. Diagnostic investigations, which may also help to determine

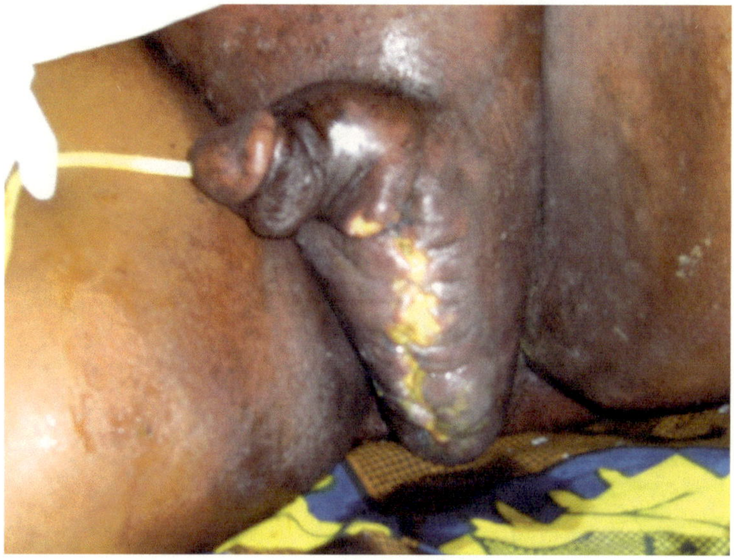

Fig. 4. Fournier's gangrene of scrotum following orchidectomy for prostate cancer. (Note fungal infection of perineal skin)

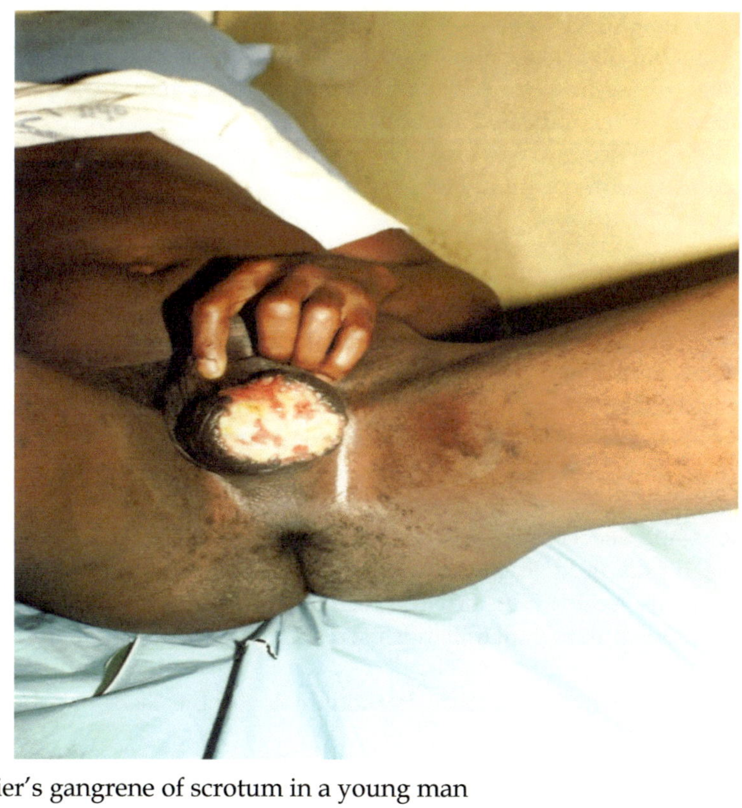

Fig. 5. Fournier's gangrene of scrotum in a young man

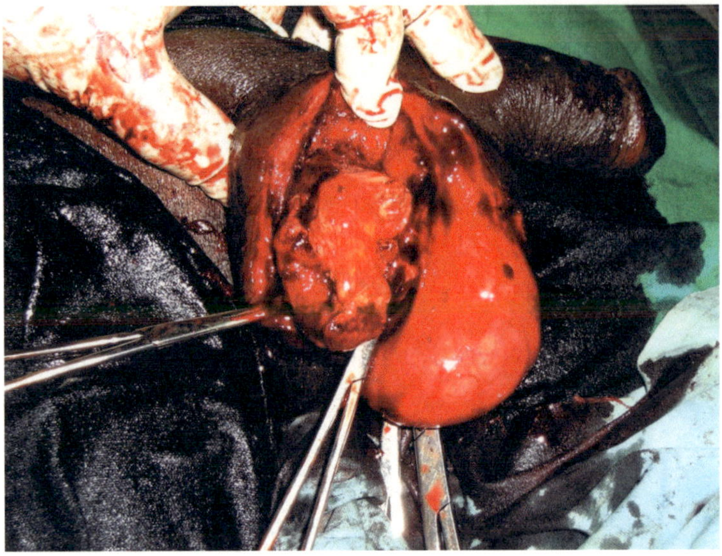

Fig. 6. Debridement for Fournier's gangrene showing healthy testes

the extent of the disease employ radiological tools such as ultra-sound scan (USS), computerised tomographic (CT) scan and magnetic resonance imaging (MRI) [16]. The hallmark in all imaging modalities is the demonstration of air in the soft tissue planes [17]. These tools may be employed when they are available. Histopathology assessment has been reported by authors but describes pathological consequences of the disease. Marjolin's ulcer has been reported to arise from the scar of a FG many years after successful treatment [18,19]. Follow up and biopsy when indicated are necessary.
Some investigations are necessary to identify the source of sepsis in FG. Thus, there may be need for cystoscopy, colonoscopy and biopsies [20].

11. Treatment

The treatment of FG depends on the status of the patient at presentation. Immediate treatment following diagnosis or suspicion includes resuscitative measures such as rehydration, blood transfusion, electrolyte replacements, multiple therapy antimicrobial agents, Oxygen and adequate analgesia [21].
Triple antimicrobial therapy is started empirically to cover aerobes and anaerobes as well as gram-negative and gram-positive organisms pending the result of microbial microscopy, culture and sensitivity from pus and or blood specimens. The organisms invariably cultured from FG include staphylococci and streptococci, coliforms, pseudomonas, bacteroides and clostridia [22]. Penicillin is used to cover streptococci while metronidazole is given against anaerobes such as bacteroides. A broad spectrum antimicrobial agent, preferably the cephalosporins combined with gentamicin is used against gram negative organisms such as the coliforms.
Sepsis leading to multiple organ failure is thought to be the leading cause of death in Fournier's gangrene [23-25].
Some authors[10,26] have doubted whether antimicrobial agents are responsible for the reduction in mortality.

The use of unprocessed honey has been advocated by clinicians reporting good outcome [27,28]. Honey inhibits bacterial growth due to its low pH, high viscosity, the hygroscopic effect and presence of inhibine and anti-oxidants [29].
Hyperbaric oxygen (HBO) was used in the erroneous belief that the crepitus in FG was of clostridial aetiology [30]. The efficacy of hyperbaric oxygen is applicable in clostridial and nonclostridial infections [30,31]. HBO increases the oxygen tension in tissues to a level that is inhibitory and lethal to anaerobic bacteria, while limiting necrosis and enhancing demarcation of gangrene [30-33]. However in a review of 42 patients with FG and in whom half were given HBO and another half not given, there was a higher mortality among the HBO patients [34]. This had been observed 10 years earlier [35].
Adequate nutrition is an essential part of treatment of FG. Enteral feeding is preferred to parenteral feeding.
Patients with co-morbid or predisposing factors need these factors controlled. In one study, the authors concluded that diabetes control was an important prognostic measure [36].
Surgical treatment is the cornerstone of the treatment of FG. A mortality of 100% has been recorded in patients with necrotizing fascitis treated without surgery [24,37,38]. Surgical treatment includes excision of all necrotic tissues. This may be repeated as necrosis is observed.
Orchidectomy may be required for testicular gangrene, a rare complication of FG. It has also been done when there was not enough scrotum to house the testis.
Reconstruction may be required to restore function and cosmetic appearance. Procedures that have been carried out vary from secondary closure of well granulated wound to flap procedures to create a neo-scrotum. The testis may be buried in inner aspect of thighs or inguinal regions temporarily, to prevent desiccation until the wound becomes clean.
In a report of FG in 10 women, the authors concluded that colostomy was an integral part of the management of FG patients requiring extensive debridement [39].
Urinary diversion via a suprapubic cystostomy is indicated in FG of the penis.
The consensus appears to be that the use of catheterization or colostomy should be pragmatic and should be decided on individual merit [28,37].

12. Complications

An uncomplicated Fournier's gangrene is one which is localized and resolves with the basic treatments of debridement, dressings and antimicrobial agents.
Morbidity includes variable periods of hospitalization with its attendant problems such as deep vein thrombosis and pulmonary embolism.
Complicated FG is found in those patients with systemic involvement including renal, pulmonary and cardiac derangements. Complicated FG may require urgent and vigorous resuscitation in the intensive care unit and reconstructive procedures. Specific complications include auto-amputation of the penis [20], fatal overwhelming sepsis, tetanus [40] and Marjolin's ulcer long after the wound has healed [41]. The testis may become gangrenous from FG in which sepsis has originated from the retroperitoneal space or the abdomen [42,43]. Scrotal skin loss may be severe not to accommodate the testis. Orchidectomy has been done for this reason [44,45]. Infertilty is a rare complication of Fournier's gangrene [46].

13. Treatment outcome

Although more patients survive from FG than die from it, the mortality in FG remains high ranging from 3 to 45% [28,47]. In a review of 1726 cases from 1950 to 1999 worldwide, reported in the English literature, the mortality rate was 16 per cent [6]. In a subsequent unpublished study of 3297 cases of FG from 1950 to 2007, the mortality rate rose to 21.1%. This is in spite of advances in technology and medical practice. It was paradoxically observed in both studies the mortality was higher in the advanced countries of America, Canada and Europe than in the underdeveloped countries.

Factors associated with high mortality include an anorectal source, advanced age, diabetes mellitus, extensive disease (involving abdominal wall or thighs), shock or sepsis at presentation, renal failure, and hepatic dysfunction [5]. Death usually results from systemic illnesses, such as sepsis, coagulopathy, diabetic ketoacidosis, acute renal failure or multiple organ failure.

14. Prognosis

Many factors impact on the prognosis in FG. Early presentation in good functional status together with adequate and prompt treatment lead to a good outcome. Co-morbid factors include older age, poorly controlled diabetes mellitus [24,48], and colorectal source of infection. Locally involved FG is associated with reduced mortality. Involvement extending beyond 5% of the body surface area portends a poor prognosis [49]. There is currently no consensus on the use of indices for predicting mortality. However, if there has been lower limb or abdominal wall involvement there is a noticeable increase in mortality rate.

There have been efforts to assess the risk of death in the disease. Laor et al. developed the Fournier's Gangrene Severity Index (FGSI) for prognostication in order to assist physicians in predicting mortality probability in FG. A severity index above 9 indicates a 75% mortality probability while under 9 indicates a 78% survival probability [50].

Other efforts to assess the risk of death in the disease have been reported [46,51]. Villanueva Saenz *et al* 2002 [52] employed APACHE II and found that patients with scores of 20 or more had a higher mortality than those with a lower score. The addition of platelet count and BSA to the variables to modify Laor's FGSIS has been claimed to improve the predictive value of FGSIS [72].

15. References

[1] Smith GL, Bunker CB, Dinneen MD. Fournier's gangrene. Br J Urol 1998; 81:347-55.

[2] Wilson B. Necrotizing fasciitis. Am Surg 1952; 18:416-431.

[3] Stephens BJ, Lathrop JC, Rice WT, Gruenberg JC. Fournier's gangrene: Historic (1764-1978) versus contemporary (1979-1988) differences in etiology and clinical importance. Am Surg 1993; 59: 149-154.

[4] Corman JM. Classic articles in colonic and rectal surgery. Dis Colon Rectum 1988; 31: 984 -988.

[5] Eke N. Fournier's gangrene: a review of 1726 cases. Br J Surg 2000; 87:718 -728.

[6] Paty R, Smith AD. Gangrene and Fournier's gangrene. Urol Clin North Am 1992; 19:149-162.

[7] Ndirika SC, Melville R, Green J. Fournier's gangrene in a man who was HIV-positive with a high CD4 count: an unusual presentation of a complex recto-scrotal fistula. Uro Today Int J 2010;10:3834.

[8] The muscles and fasciae of the pelvis. Bartleby.com edition of Gray's Anatomy of the human body Chapter 6.

[9] Clayton MD, Fowler JE Jr, Sharifi R, Pearl RK. Causes, presentation and survival of fifty-seven patients with necrotizing fasciitis of the male genitalia. Surg Gynecol Obstet 1990 ; 170: 49-55.

[10] Mergenhagen SE, Thonard JC, Scherp HW. Studies on synergistic infections. Experimental infections with anaerobic streptococci. J Infect Dis 1958 ; 103:33-44.

[11] Meleney FL. Hemolytic Streptococcus gangrene. Arch Surg 1924; 9:317-321.

[12] Ben-Aharon U, Borenstein A, Eisenkraft S, Lifschitz O, Leviav A. Extensive necrotizing soft tissue infection of the perineum. Isr J Med Sci 1996; 32:745-749.

[13] Basoglu M, Gül O, Yildirgan I, Balik AA, Ozbey I, Oren D. Fournier's gangrene: review of fifteen cases. Am Surg1997; 63:1019-1021.

[14] Goyette M. Group A streptococcal necrotizing fasciitis Fournier's gangrene - Quebec Can Commun Dis Rep 1997; 23:101-103.

[15] Yoneda A, Fujita F, Tokai H, Ito Y, Haraguchi M, Tajima Y, Kanematsu T. MRI can determine the adequate area for debridement in the case of Fournier's gangrene. Int Surg 2010; 95:76-79.

[16] Levenson RB, Singh AK, Novelline RA. Fournier gangrene: role of imaging. Radiographics. 2008; 28:519-528.

[17] Schneider PR, Russele RC, Zoog EG. Fournier's gangrene: a general surgery problem. World J Surg 1983; 7: 288–294.

[18] Chintamani, Shankar M, Singhal V, Singh JP, Bansal A, Saxena S. Squamous cell carcinoma developing in the scar of Fournier's gangrene Case report. BMC Cancer. 2004; 4:16.

[19] Eke N, Onwuchekwa AC. Fournier's gangrene of the penis associated with adenocarcinoma of the rectum and diabetes mellitus. Acta Urologica Italica 1999; 13:207-209.

[20] Ong HS, Ho YH. Genitoperineal gangrene: experience in Singapore. Aust N Z J Surg 1996; 66:291-293.

[21] Laucks SS II. Fournier's gangrene. Surg Clin North Am 1994; 74:1339 -1352.

[22] Cohen M, Tamir E, Abu-Abid S, Galili Y, Giladi M, Avital S, Shafir R,Klausner Y. [The diagnosis and treatment of Fournier's gangrene]. Harefuah 1998; 135: 360 -363, 407

[23] Yanar H, Taviloglu K, Ertekin C, Guloglu R, Zorba U, Cabioglu N, Baspinar I. Fournier's gangrene: risk factors and strategies for management. World J Surg 2006; 30:1750-1754.

[24] Adinolfi MF, Voros DC, Moustouskas NM, Hardin WD, Nichols RL. Severe systemic sepsis resulting from neglected perineal infections. South Med J 1983; 76: 746-749.

[25] Adams JR Jr, Mata JA, Venable DD, Culkin DJ, Bocchini JA Jr. Fournier's gangrene in children. Urology 1990; 35:439-441.

[26] Effem SE. Recent advances in the management of Fournier' gangrene: preliminary observations. Surgery 1993; 113:2000-2004.

[27] Hejase MJ, Simonin JE, Bihrle R, Coogan CL. Fournier's gangrene: experience with 38 patients. Urology 1996; 47: 734-739.

[28] Moore OA, Smith LA, Campbell F, Seers K, McQuay HJ, Moore RA. Systematic review of the use of honey as a wound dressing. BMC Complement Alternat Med 2001; 1:2-8.

[29] Korhonen K, Hirn M, Niinikoski J. Hyperbaric oxygen in the treatment of Fournier's gangrene. Eur J Surg 1998; 164:251-255.

[30] Hollabaugh RS Jr, Dmochowski RR, Hickerson WL, Cox CE. Fournier's gangrene: therapeutic impact of hyperbaric oxygen. Plast Reconstr Surg 1998; 101:94–100.

[31] Benizri E, Fabiani P, Migliori G. Gangrene of the perineum. Urology 1996; 47:935-939.

[32] Ziser A, Girski Z, Gozal D, Melamed Y, Adler M. Hyperbaric oxygen therapy for Fournier's gangrene. Crit Care Med 1985;13:773–774.
[33] Mindrup SR, Kealey GP, Fallon B. Hyperbaric oxygen for the treatment of Fournier's gangrene. J Urol 2005; 173:1975-1977.
[34] Shupak A, Shoshani O, Goldenberg I, et al. Necrotizing fasciitis: an indication for hyperbaric oxygenation Surgery 1995; 118:873–878.
[35] Malik AM, Sheikh S, Pathan R, Khan A, Sheikh U. The spectrum of presentation and management of Fournier's gangrene-an experience of 73 cases. J Pak Med Assoc 2010; 60:617-619.
[36] Flanigan RC, Kursch FD, Mc Dougal WS, Persky L. Synergistic gangrene of the scrotum and penis secondary to colorectal disease. J Urol 1978; 119:369.
[37] Okeke LI. Fournier's gangrene in Ibadan. Afr J Med Med Sci 2000; 29:323–324.
[38] Hasdemir AO, Büyükaşik O, Cöl C. The clinical characteristics of female patients with Fournier's gangrene. Int Urogynecol J Pelvic Floor Dysfunct. 2009; 20:1439-1443.
[39] Omotoso AB, Aderibigbe A. Fournier's gangrene complicated by tetanus: case report. Orient J Med 1990; 2: 207–208.
[40] Schneider PR, Russell RC, Zook EG. Fournier's gangrene of the penis: a report of two cases. Ann Plast Surg 1986; 17:87-90.
[41] Gerber MP, Peterson NE. Scrotal gangrene. Urology 1973; 1:466-469.
[42] Klutke CG, Miles BJ, Obeid E. Unusual presentation of sigmoid diverticulitis as an acute scrotum. J Urol 1988; 139:380-381.
[43] Tripathi FM, Khanna NN, Venkateshwarlu V, Sinha JK. Gangrene of the scrotum: a series of 20 cases. Br J Plast Surg 1978; 31:242–243.
[44] Patel A, Ramsay JW, Whitfield HN. Fournier's gangrene of the scrotum following day care vasectomy. J R Soc Med 1991; 84:49-50.
[45] Baskin LS, Carroll PR, Cattolica EV, McAninch JW. Necrotising soft tissue infections of the perineum and genitalia. Bacteriology, treatment and risk assessment. Br J Urol 1990; 65:524-529.
[46] Spirnak JP, Resnick MI, Hampel N, Persky L. Fournier's gangrene: report of 20 patients. J Urol 1984; 131:289-291.
[47] Moorthy K, Rao PP, Supe AN. Necrotising perineal infection: a fatal outcome of ischiorectal fossa abscesses. J R Coll Surg Edinb 2000; 45:281-284.
[48] Palmer LS, Winter HI, Tolia BM, Reid RE, Laor E. Surgical debridement on survival in Fournier's gangrene. Br J Urol 1995; 76: 208-212.
[49] Laor E, Palmer LS, Tolia BM, Reid RE, Winter HI. Outcome prediction in patients with Fournier's gangrene. J Urol 1995; 154:89-92.
[50] Asci R, Sarikaya S, Buyukalpelli R, Yilmaz AF, Yildiz S. Fournier's gangrene: risk assessment and enzymatic debridement with lyophilized collagenase application. Eur Urol 1998; 34: 411-418.
[51] Villanueva-Saenz E, Martinez Hernandez-Magro P, Valdes Ovalle M, Montes Vega J, Alvarez-Tostado F JF. Experience in management of Fournier's gangrene. Tech Coloproctol 2002; 6: 5-13.
[52] Samad A. Predictive value of modified severity index for Fournier's gangrene. J Liaquat Uni Med Health Sci 2007; 6: 16-20.

5

Fournier's Gangrene – Medical and Surgical Considerations

Oscar Estrada Ferrer
Consorci Sanitari del Maresme,
Colorectal Surgery,
Mataró. Barcelona
Spain

1. Introduction

There is a consensus to consider Founier's Gangrene a form of necrotizing fascitis that typically starts in the perineal region, but can involves to genital, perianal or surroundings structures. Although is typically described in men, it can also affect women and, very rarely, children.

A synergistic infective process is allways present triggering to thrombosis of the subcutaneous blood vessels, developing a gangrene of the skin and later of deeper nearby tissues. Local edema and specially hypoxia affects local blood supply. This situation offers an ideal medium for growth to aerobic and anaerobic bacteria, and sometimes causing typical crepitation.

The local process is associated with severe systemic manifestations usually related to endotoxin liberation Rapidly dispersion of the infection may cause the death of the patient up to 45% of cases.

2. Historical considerations

In 1883, Jean Alfred Founier described a scrotal necrotizing fasciitis in five youngs males previously sane. In the initial Fournier's description, the illness was considered idiopatic. However, in 1764 Bauriene reported a case of scrotal gangrene, witch is considered to be the fisrt case published in medical literature, although the origin of the case was not idiopathic but due to injury by ox horn. (Medina Polo et al., 2009)

In the past, some authors advocated that the eponym Fournier should be reserved for the idiophatic cases of perineal gangrene, and use the term secondary necrotizing fasciitis to the cases with a proven etiology. In fact this classification is not used in the present (Eke, 2000)

The american surgeon Frank L. Meleney described in 1924 for the first time the importance of extensive debridement of the necrotic tissues to achieve better results. The term Meleney's gangrene is associated with a synergistic gangrene that affects the skin and subcutaneous tissues, but not the deep fascia except in advanced cases, and always stars as a necrotic ulcer (Meleney, 1924) Other historical terms applied to Forunerir's Gangrene include periurethral phlegmon, phagedema or synergistic necrotizing cellulitis.

3. Aethilogy

3.1 Anatomical origin

Far from being idiopathic, the origin of the process can be located in one of these three sites: Lost of cutaneous barrier of perineal skin, urinary tract or intestinal tract. Recent studies conclude that only in a small percentage of the cases is not possible to determine the origin of the sepsis. The importance of the sources are variable according to the authors. Possibly the urogenital origin is the most important of all, followed by the anorectal and the cuteneous in the last position.

3.1.1 Urogenital origin

Any surgery or non-surgical procedure on the urogenital territory like vasectomy, urethral catheterization, penile prosthetic implants, prostate biopsies and others could be the gateway of the germs.

Accidental local traumatism are described to be origin of the sepsis.

Also any local infection as epididymitis, chronic urinary tract infection or predisposing factors as neurogenic bladder could be the etiology of the disease.

Urethral stricture is one of the main predisposing factor, with incidence ranging up to 31%. In theory, urethral stricture may lead to urethral diverticula and its eventual rupture could induce urine extravasation. In these situation, the leak of contaminaded urine is the origin of Founier´s gangrene. (Hakan Yanar et al, 2006)

In women, additional causes of Fournier gangrene have included septic abortion, episiotomy, and hysterectomy, but in case of genital gangrene the physician always has to look for a vulvar Bartholin's abscess as responsible of the process up to 24% of cases. (Eke, 2000)

3.1.2 Anorectal origin

Hidden perianal abscess is certainly the main cause of gangrene in this region. Other reasons like colorectal surgical procedures, have also been described. The most referrals are haemorroidal interventions, carcinoma of the colon and rectum and diverticulits

Traumatic local wounds or anal intercourse appear to be possible aethiologic factors (Smith et al., 1998)

3.1.3 Cutaneous origin

From the original description of the ox horn penetrating wound of Bauriene in the XVIII century, any possible traumatism in the perineal region are described as origin of the septic process. Animal or human bites, burns, piercings, injections are only an example of possible causes.

3.1.4 Idiophatic origin

As I has been stated above, currently idiopathic origin is a lower percentage of cases. More extensive cultures with better conditions of collection and grown, make possible to identify in most cases the germ responsible and indirectly the anatomical origin.

In some series neither the identification of the causative organism nor localizing the source to genitourinary or colorectal origin was associated with high mortality. (Corcoran et al., 2008)

3.2 Involved organism

These organism are usual commensals of perineal skin and genital organs, and include Clostridia, Klebsiella, Streptococci, Coliforms, Staphylococci, Bacteriodes and Corynebacteria. Characteristically in Founier's Gangrene exists synergism between theoretically low aggressive bacteries alone.
In this situation of synergism, one bacterium produces a nutrient for another, witch produces leucocidal toxin. This toxin then protects both organism from phagocytosis. Similarly, the aerobic bacteria consume the oxygen present in tissues that benefits the growth of anaerobic. (Eke, 2000)

3.2.1 Most frequent isolation in cultures

The most commonly isolated aerobic microorganism are Escherichia coli, Klebsiella pneumoniae and Staphylococcus aureus. The most commonly isolated anaerobic microorganism is Bacteriodes fragilis. (Patty et al., 1992) Actually both aerobes and anaerobes are present in the tissues but anaerobes are less frequent isolated because these samples are more difficult to preserve. In some series, a mean of four different organisms is cultured from each patient. (Addison et al. 1984)

Gram Positive	Gram negative
Staphylococcus aureus	Escherichia coli
Enterecoccus species	Pseudomona aeruginosa
Streptococcus species	Proteus
	Acinetobacter
	Klebsiella species
	Enterobacter species
	Bacteriodes

Table 1. Isolation from tissue cultures. Shown in order of detection (Yanar et al., 2006)

While aerobic bacteria often cause platelet aggregation, anaerobes are able to produce heparinase. Both organism tend to activate intravascular clotting. These effects are fundamental to the onset of vascular thrombosis and dermal gangrene.
Microorganisms causing gangrene also release a variety of proteins that have the capacity to destroy tissue directly.
Gram negative bacteria such as E. coli, Proteus and Klebsiella are known to produce lipopolysaccaride endotoxin also implicated in thrombosis of small vessels. Streptococci and Staphylo segregate hyaluronidase driving to to connective tissue necrosis. Some anaerobic organism also produce hydrogen and nitrogen which accumulate in the tissues causing crepitus.
Thus a destructive infection results from a combination of relatively nonpathogenic bacteria. Patient's immunosuppression could in most cases worse the processes. (Smith et al., 1998)

4. Predisposing factors

The common denominator in all these patients is impaired host resistance from reduced cellular immunity

4.1 Age and sex

Although the description of Fournier's Gangrene is done in young patients and males, it is increasingly evident that the disease affects elderly people and women also. In most studies the ratio between males and female is 10:1 (Eke, 2000)

The usual form of presentation is men between 50 and 70 years, with one or more predisposing factors. From early studies in the mid-twentieth century, the average age likely to present the clinical picture has been increasing. In 1945 the average age was 40.9 years and currently ranges between 50 and 70 years.

At present as opposed to what was believed at the time of Fournier, it is accepted that children may be affected by the disease. (Montoya et al., 2009). More than fifty cases have been reporded until today. Due to the usual absence of predisposing factors in children some reports have indicated a better prognosis in this patients. Debridement in this cases need to be radical too. In the pediatric literature there is description of healing with limited excision of scrotal afection. (Ameh et al., 2004)

4.2 Diabetes mellitus

It is considered the most frequent predisposing factor. Presence of Diabetes mellitus has been reported as 39%-64% of patients with Fournier's Gangrene in different reviews

Hyperglycemia has been found to have detrimental effects on cellular immunity.

Theoretically, decreased phagocytic activity and neutrophil dysfunction typically presented in diabetic patients could be associated with more progressive fatal outcome. Although numerous review articles have failed to demonstrate this item. (Korkut et al., 2003)

4.3 Chronic alcoholism

Chronic alcoholism is the second predisposing factor, according to some authors. In others publications, is considered the most prevalent factor (Smith et al., 1998)

4.4 Other factors

Exists a large number of factors that can be associated with the disease. Liver diseases, Malignancy, Obesity, HIV, leukemia, are just one example of diseases, all with some degree of alteration of the immune system

5. Clinical presentation

5.1 Symptoms and physical findings. Pain as most common presentation. Keys for clinical suspicion

The most common presentation was perianal or scrotal pain.

Systemic signs and symptoms are often associated to systemic inflammatory response syndrome (SIRS). Any patient suffering from gangrene could present fever, tachycardia, leucocytosis or tachypnea, We consider severe sepsis if there is dysfunction of one organ, hypotension or hypoperfusion.

In early stages, patients often have systemic symptoms of sepsis which appear disproportionate to appearance of the perineal-scrotal skin. (Smith et al., 1998)

Besides pain, other local symptoms are swelling,, purulent discharge from the perineum or crepitus. (Ersay et al., 2007)

It is very important to consider the strict control of all patients with perianal pain and no external lesion detected, because it could be the initial phase of the disease. The velocity of fascial necrosis has been noted to be as 2-3 cm per hour, making early diagnosis crucial(Safioleas et al., 2006)

In contrast to the typical scrotal involvement, testicular involvement is rare. The blood supply to the scrotum comes from the pudendal arteries, while testicular artery is a direct branch from aorta. When testicular involvement occurs, it indicates a possible intra-abdominal source of infection.

Crepitus in gangrenous tissues gives the false impression of clostridial infection. Nevertheless, the gas-gangrene organism Clostridium perfringens, has occasionally been isolated.

Gas production was demonstrated by the finding of crepitus (cellulitis crackling) may be due to the presence of this anaerobic microorganisms or facultative anaerobes like Escherichia coli.

Cellulitis
Strangulated hernia
Scrotal abscess
Herpes simplex
Gonococcal infections
Pyoderma Gangrenosum
Vasculitis
Local traumatism

Table 2. Main differential diagnosis of Fournier's Gangrene. (Smith et al., 1998)

The importance of recognizing patients who have vasculitis or pyoderma gangrenosum is that optimal treatment of these diseases is the opposite of Fournier's Gangrene., because they need high doses of corticosteroids.

In summary the key to diagnosis is the presence of pain in perineal region and rapid local changes associated with systemic symptoms, that often seems in many cases excessive in relation to the initial findings.

5.2 Laboratory findings

In a large retroscpective study of 68 patients, Corcoran et al. described significant differences between non survivors and survivals in admission laboratory parameters such as high serum Creatinine, lactate and calcium or low bicarbonate. Increased calcium in serum may be due to renal failure, bacteriemia or use of parenteral nutrition. (Corcoran et al., 2008)

Clayton et al reported that BUN level (UREA) >50 mg/dL was statistically significant for mortality among the parameters.

Creatinine, hematocrit, hemoglobin and alkaline phosphatase levels correladed with a worse prognosis in non survival group.

Some studies have demonstrated that admission hypomagnesaemia is associated with high mortality in critical ill patients. Reduced intestinal absorption, increased urinay losses or intracellular shift are possible reasons of this action. Monitoring serum magnesium levels in patients with Fournier's Gangrene might have prognostic and therapeutic implications and is used today in specialized groups. (Erol at al., 2010)

5.3 Severity Index. FGSI

In a study published by Laor et al. was described for the first time a Fournier's gangrene severity index (FGSI) along the lines of the Acute Physiologiy and Chronic Health Evaluation score (APACHE II). They identified several prognostic factors associated with a worse prognosis.

The FGSI score were calculated twice, at the time of admission and at the time of discharge or death.

Physiological variable					Normal				
	+4	+3	+2	+1	0	+1	+2	+3	+4
Temperature	>41	>39		38.5-38.9	36-38.4	34-35.9	32-33.9	<31.9	<29.9
Heart rate	>180	140-179	110-139		70-109		55-69	40-54	<39
Respiratory rate	>50	35-49		25-34	12-24	10-11	6-9		<5
Na	>180	160-179	155-159	150-154	130-149		120-129	111-119	<110
K+	>7	6-6.9		5.5-5.9	3.5-5.4	3-3.4	2.5-2.9		<2.5
Creatinine	>3.5	2-3.4	1.5-1.9		0.6-1.4		<0.6		
Hematocrit	>60		50-59.9	46-49.9	30-45.9		20-29.9		<20
Leucocytes	>40		20-39.9	15-19.9	3-14.9		1-2.9		<1
Bicarbonate	>52	41-51.9		32-40.9	22-31.9		18-21.9	15-17.9	<15

Table 3. Fournier's Gangrene Severity Index

In the FGSI score, nine parameters were calculated, temperature, heart rate, respiratory rate, serum sodium, potassium,. Creatinine, bicarbonate levels, hematocrite and leukocyte. The degree of derivation from normal is graded from 0 to 4. The individual values are summed to obtain the FGSI score. (Laor et al., 1995)
Results published in the articles shows that a score >9 has 75% of death and patients with a score <9 were associated with 78% of survival.
Other series of patients analyzed with the same score shows FGSI >10.5 is associated with 96% of death and <10.5 96% of survival. (Kabay et al. 2008)
Other medical groups use Chalson Comorbidity Index (useful not only in case of Founier's Gangrene). It was calculated using 17 weighted indicators of coexisting conditions. A high score in Chalson Comorbidity Index is associated with a high mortality. (Erol et al., 2010)

5.4 Pathways of disease spread

Perineal anatomy and its fascial planes could be compared with. two triangles: the anal triangle and the urogenital triangle The anal triangle is posterior to the line that crosses the ischial tuberosities, instead the urogenital triangle is anterior to this line. Infection arising from the anal triangle can spread along the
Colles fascia and progress anteriorly along the Dartos fascia to involve the scrotum and penis. It can also pass superiorly to involve the anterior abdominal wall.
Buttocks and thighs may be affected if the infection goes beyond the barrier of Colles fascia.
Infection originating from the urogenital triangle, can initially involve the ventral aspect of the penis. If infection is not initially treated it may progress as I wrote before. (Levenson et al., 2008)

5.5 Radiological explorations. Role of X-ray exploration

Although the diagnosis of Fournier gangrene is most commonly made clinically, CT can be used in doubtful cases or to assess the extent of involvement.
Presence of collections, subcutaneous emphysema and its extent, including retroperitoneal extension, are well evaluated at CT. Actually, CT has greater specificity for evaluating disease extent than does any other radiological exploration or physical examination
In early Fournier gangrene, CT can show small bubbles in the subcutaneous tissues, that has not yet been detected by physical examination.
Post treatment follow-up CT could be used to determine improvement or worsening of disease and schedule additional surgery interventions
In any case, a radiological exploration is not a justification for surgical delay if the clinical suspicion is present.
Ultrasonography is also useful in differential diagnosis with others entities as presence of gas gangrene from inguinoscrotal incarcerated hernia;
Soft-tissue air is also more obvious at US than at radiography. In ultrasonography evidence of gas within the scrotal wall may be seen prior to clinical crepitus (Levenson et al., 2008)

6. Treatment

6.1 Medical treatment

6.1.1 Prompt resuscitation of the patient. Fluid therapy

In the first phase of the disease is essential to maintain the patient's hemodynamic stability, providing fluid therapy with crystalloids. Some groups also managed these septic patients with colloids like albumin that seems to improve haemodynamics.

If necessary, begin with vasoactive drugs in the emergency room.

6.1.2 Broad spectrum antibiotics coverage

Antibiotic treatment alone will not cure in any case this disease.
Recommendations of published guidelines are based on low levels of scientific evidence, hence the difficulty to agree on a single therapeutic strategy.
Empiric broad-spectrum antibiotic thereapy should be instituted as soon as possible, until the culture results could make adjusted the therapy
The antibiotic regimen chosen must have a high degree of effectiveness against sthylococcal and streptococcal bacteria, gram-negative, coliforms, pseudomona, bacteroides and clostridium. (Laucks, 1994) Classically Triple therapy is usually recommended. Third generation cefhalosporins or aminoglycosides, plus penicillin and metronidazole.
Sometimes if we doubt of the possible origin of the sepsis and a streptococcal toxic syndrome could cause the clinical symptoms, we should associated clindamycin and penicillin to the antibiotic therapy
The reason is that clindamycin in vitro studies demonstrated both toxin suppression and modulation of cytokine production (Stevens et al., 2005)
Clindamycine always should be administrated in association, because is described a high percentage of resistances of Bacteroides.

6.1.3 New antibiotics strategies

New clinical guidelines currently recommend the use of Carbapenems (Imipenem, meropenem, ertapenem) or piperaziline-tazobactam.
Tigecycline is a macrolid related antibiotic that could be a good alternative in penicilline allergies patients
These therapies have good antibacterial spectrum, a large volume of distribution and lower renal toxicity compared with the aminoglycoside.
This new trend suggest that classically triple therapy could be replaced in certain circunstances for the use of new generation antibiotics.(Jimeno et al., 2010)
If there are risk factors for colonization by resistant bacteria (previous hospital admission, prior prolonged antibiotic treatment, institutionalization), we recommended adding therapy to linezolid or Daptomicine (Stevens et al., 2005)

6.2 Fournier's Gangrene: A surgical emergency

6.2.1 Radical surgical debridement. Early aggressive treatment that saves lives

It is widely recommend a debridement of the necrotic tissue as soon as possible
(Laor et al. 1995) found no significant difference between the onset time of symptoms, early surgical treatment and mortality, but others studies from (kabay et al. 2008) and (Korkut et al. 2003) shows that this time interval should be as short as possible.
Asfar et al. reported that insufficient debridements results in increased mortality. However, repeated aggressive debridements with one or two days intervals have resulted in reduced mortalily rates (Kabay et al., 2008)
The actual relationship between the lesion size of Fournier gangrene and the final survival is still controversial.
Debridement of deep fascia and muscle is not usually required as these areas are rarely involved similar to testes. Debridement should be stopped when separation of the skin and the subcutaneous is not perform easily, because the cutaneous necrosis is not a good marker.

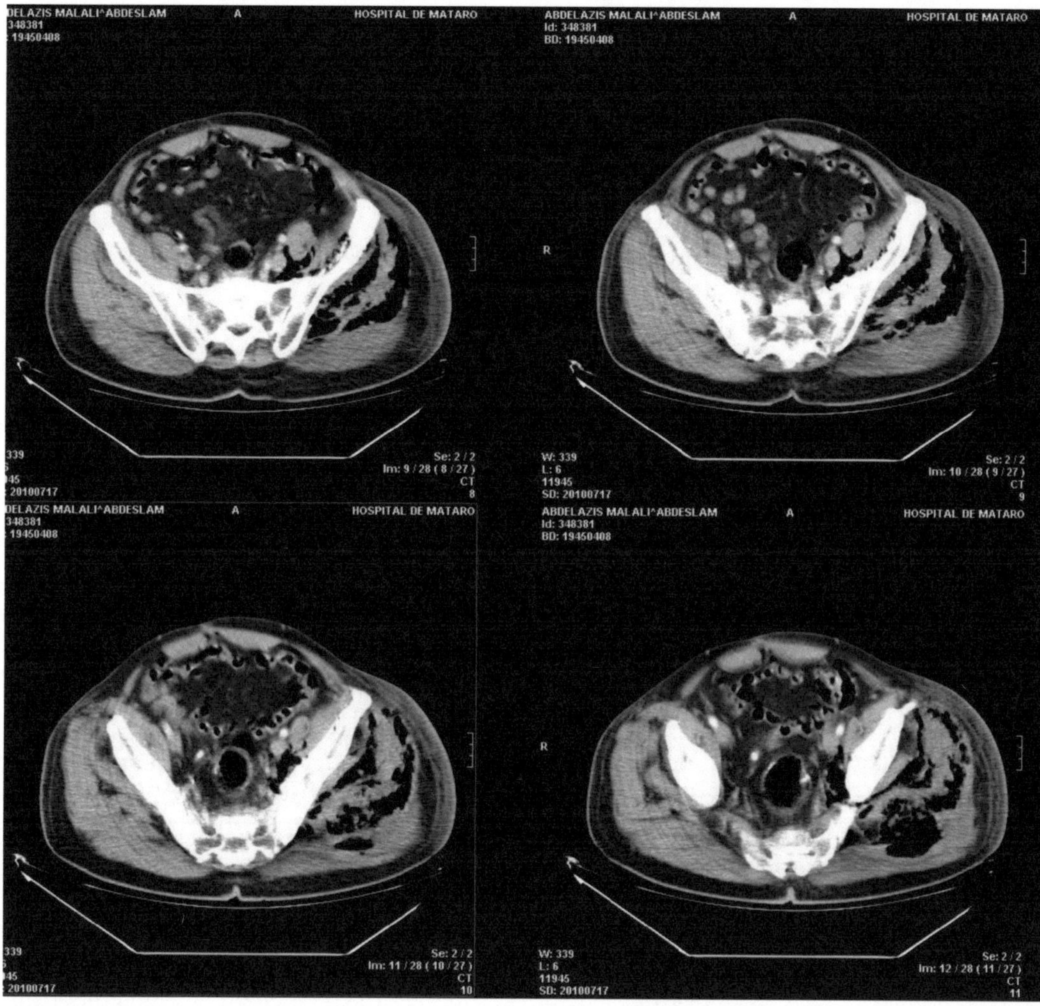

Fig. 1. CT-Scan showing gas in gluteus and in the retroperitoneal space in a 66 years old patient with ascendant Fournier's Gangrene (Author's image)

In some series orchiectomy was performed because of observed severe infection in peritesticular tissues, although in the pathological review the testicles were not found to be involved(Yanar et al., 2006)

It is possible to temporally place the testes into subcutaneous pouch until healing or reconstruction complete (Smith et al. 1998)

Penectomy was required only in very isolated cases. (Corman et al. 1999)

6.2.2 Role of hyperbaric oxygen therapy

Hyperbaric oxygen therapy implies placing the patient in a environment of increased ambient pressure while breathing 100% oxygen, resulting in enhanced oxygenation of the arterial blood and tissues. (Wilkinson & Doolette, 2004)

In vitro demonstrated benefits of hyperbaric oxygen include adequate oxygenation for optimal neutrophil phagocytic function, inhibition of anaerobic growth, increased fibroblast proliferation and angiogenesis, reduction of edema by vasoconstriction and increased intracellular antibiotics transportation.

Hypoxia may also reduce the effectiveness of several antibiotics (vancomycin, ciprofloxacine) while hyperoxia may help others. For example aminoglycosides cross the cell membrane of the microorganism by an oxygen-depenent pump In addition, some side effects has been described as toxic reaction of central nervous system and barotrauma injury to the middle ear. In some cases a surgical procedure (tympanostomy tube insertion or myringotomy) should be performed prior to the hyperbaric oxygen therapy.

The use of Hyberparic Oxyegn Therpay continues to be cause of debate. Certainly no prospective controlled trials have been published for this condition. Although this treatment is supported by some small studies, hyperbaric oxygen should not delay surgical debridement. (Riseman et al. 1990)

There are 6 studies examining the effect of O2 therpay in necrotizing soft tissues infections. 4 report a significant survival advantage for patients and 2 not (Wilkinson & Doolette, 2004)

In many cases, lack of facilities to perform hyperbaric therapy makes difficult his recommendation today generally.

6.2.3 Topical therapy

Natural and unprocessed honey was used with good results in debridement areas. This antibacterial effect is considered to result from hypertonic environment and phenolics acids making and antibacterial effect.

Honey has a low pH of 3.6 and contains enzymes which digest necrotic tissues. These changes occurs within a week of applying honey to the wound. Unfortunately there is no randomized study about the efficacy of honey in this special situations. (Eke, 2000)

Application of Sodium Hypochlorite 0.5 % (Dakin's Solution) or hydrogen peroxide in the postoperative period was described with good results.

Application is justified when hydrogen peroxide is used in the correct circumstances, but but should take precautions when used in closed spaces or under pressure, where liberated oxygen cannot escape, and dangerous side effects are described as blood oxygen embolism. From the same way, hydrogen peroxide subcutaneos crepitus can be confused with typical disease progression. (SLEIGH & LINTER, 1985)

Enzymatic debridements with lypophilized collagenase application are other local treatment that have been shown to be beneficial (Aşci et al., 1998)

Use of fibrin glue has recently been suggested in skin defects with no active infection (DeCastro & Morey, 2002)

6.2.4 Local negative pressure treatment (VAC)

The vacuum assisted closure system consist of a foam dressing placed in large areas of debridement with an overlying adhesive seal to maintain the zone in subatmospheric pressure. This has been shown to reduce the local oedema increase local blood flow and improves the formation of granulation tissue. The device could be cut for better adjust in cavities or irregular wounds. It is recommended to change the device every to 2-3 days

Possible handicaps are high costs and the necessary immobilization of the patient

6.3 Fecal diversion. Colostomy vs rectal diversion devices

6.3.1 Colostomy

Performing a colostomy is a common technique in patients with extensive involvement of the perineal area for the disease. The rationale for rectal diversion includes a decrease in the number of germs in perineal region and improved wound healing. (Estrada et al., 2009)
Justification for its construction are anal sphincter involving, fecal incontinence or continues fecal contamination of the wound's margins.
In several papers, the percentage of patients with a colostomy is around 15% depending on the series.. (Yanar et al., 2006))
In contrast to the study of Corocan et al, others series reported that formation of a diverting colostomy were associated with increased mortality. (Erol et al., 2010)) Korkut et al. reported 45 cases of FG and showed that mortality among patients not requiring a stoma was 7%, but was 38% among patients in whom stoma was required.
Diverting colostomy does not eliminate the necessity of multiple debridements, nor reduces the number of these procedures. However this associated technique may lead to early oral intake and thus may help to improve the wound cure process with better nutrition and less contamination of wounds. Anyway, serious stoma- related complications were described like wound infection, stomal ischemia, and evisceration. (Akcan et al. 2009)) We must also take into account the psychological consequences of a colostomy, in a patient with extensive mutilation of his body.

6.3.2 Rectal diversion devices

The Flexi-seal Fecal Management system is a silicone catheter designed to divert fecal matter in patients with diarrhea, local burns or skin ulcers. The device protects the wounds from fecal contamination and reduces the same way that a colostomy both the risk of skin breakdown and repeated inoculation with colonic flora. We consider that in selected cases the utilization of the device can replace colostomy, with the equivalent results regarding wound healing and local infection control.
It is recommended to explore the canal anal before placement of the catheter in order to avoid rectal injuries. This device avoids complications related to stomas, including better psychological recovery of the patient and also may have an economic benefit. (Estrada et al., 2009) A formal contraindication is rectal neoplasm, penetrating rectal injuries or fistulas.
Although some authors suggest cystostomy for urinary diversion, most authors believe that urinary catheterization is sufficient for satisfactory diversion (Yanar et al., 2006)

6.4 Postoperative period in the Intensive care unit

6.4.1 Renal function

Renal failure is the most common complication in this patients, associated with hemodynamic instability and massive toxin liberation to the bloodstream. Fluid resuscitation, vasoactive drugs and in some cases hemodialysis are important components required to manage potential fatal complications like acidosis or uremia.
Administration of albumin in this septic patients, appears to improve survival in many trials.

6.4.2 Blood glucose control

Strict glucose control in the intensive care period seems to be one of the most important parameters to preserve for the optimums homeostasis of the septic patient. In some cases, insulin pump infusion is necessary to achieve this objective.

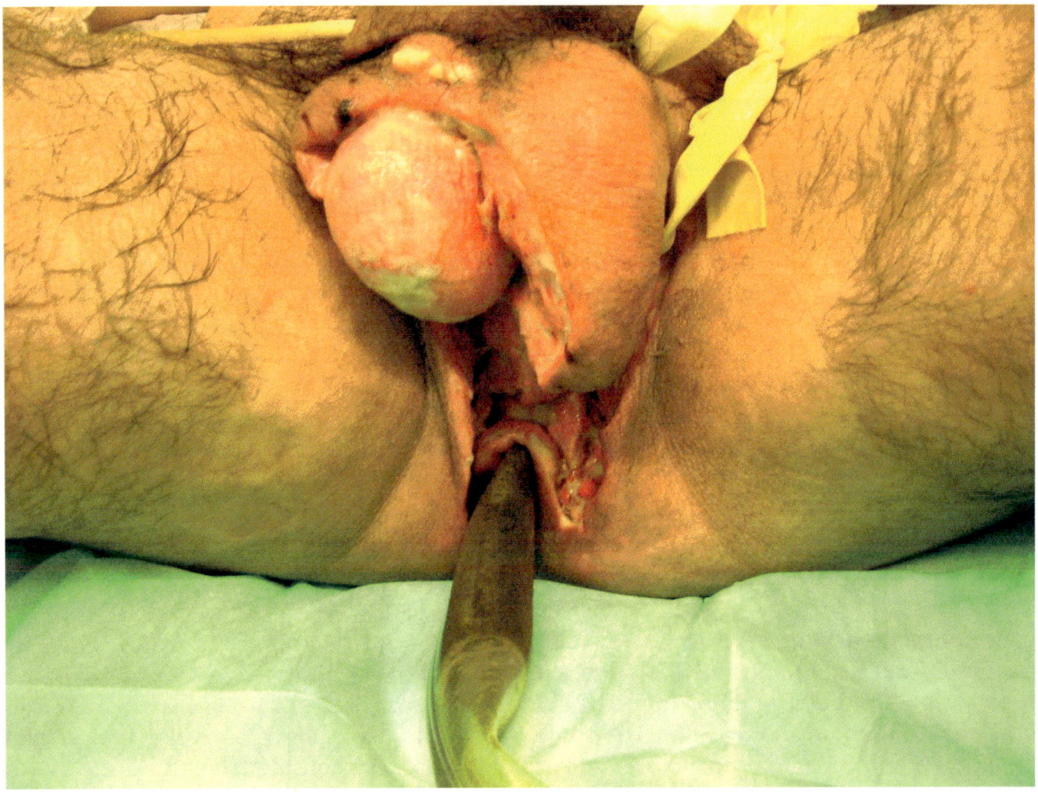

Fig. 2. Patient with Fournier's Gangrene and extensive debridement zone. See de rectal catheter placement that prevents local contamination and avoids colostomy performing. (Author's image)

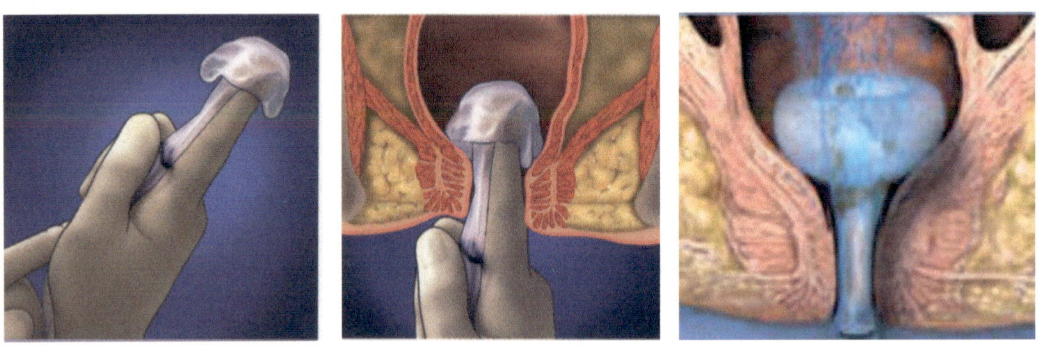

Fig. 3. Flexi seal rectal catheter placement. Rectal balloon is placed to the sphincter to prevent faecal leakage

6.4.3 Nutritional support

Physicians have long recognized that stress causes increase in basic energetic requirements in septic patients. In this population, repeated surgical procedures and mechanical ventilation decreases the possibility of oral intake. In this cases provision of nutritional support via parenteral nutrition does not assure adequate nutrient intake in a high percentage of patients. Some data shows that this critically ill population needs a provision of calories at about 125% of basal requirements (Graves et al., 2004)

This point can be achieved providing additional enteral intake.

Many articles defines.the theoretical benefit of oligoelements (like arginine, citrulline and glutamine) in the nutrition of this patients.

Plasma concentrations of L-arginine are substantially decreased in patients with sepsis and has been correlated with a worse prognosis in this population. Arginine participates in important physiological roles, including wound healing and immune function. and the arginine–NO system is essential in the regulation of vascular tone and blood pressure

However, further studies are necessary to identify the potential utility of supplementation with arginine and/or glutamine in septic patients.

6.5 Plastic surgery. The final step

There are two main strategies for reconstructive surgery, at the same time of admission (De la Cruz et al., 1996) or in a posterior period when the acute process is fully resolved. A reconstructive procedure was considered for patients presenting with an extensive healthy granulation tissue formation on the wound base

Secondary healing or delayed primary closure was applied safely for small areas.

The scrotal advancement technique was used for small sized skin defects of the scrotum.

Split-thickness skin grafts were performed in patients with a large area of skin loss, especially in the abdominal wall

Myocutaneus flap as Gracilis muscle flap is useful in some cases. Patients with a large and deep perineal defect often need this technique to eliminate the dead space. The well vascularized muscle flap demonstrates greater resistance to bacterial inoculums and in wounds with some degree of contamination.(Chen et al., 2010) Another alternative is the pudental thigh flap. It is a fasciocutaneous flap based on the terminal branches of the superficial perineal artery, which arises from the internal pudendal artery. The advantages of this flap are relatively simplicity and good blood supply. The donor site can be closed primarily and no muscle function is sacrificed.

7. High mortality rates. Still a problem in the 21st century

The mortality rate associated with Fournier'sGangrene varies from 3 to 45 %depending on the series. Although is lower than others forms of necrotizing fasciitis, probably because the scrotal area allows a relatively more efficient surgical debridement (Eke, 2000)

In this retrospective review of 45 consecutive patients, the presence of diabetes and the interval on the onset of clinical symptoms to the initial surgical intervention affected outcome in both univariate and multivariate analyses. (Korkut et al., 2003) but others studies failed in demonstrated this relation (Corcoran et al., 2008)

Idiophatic Fournier's Gangrene is not an independent additional contributory factor to the mortality in many series (Kabay et al., 2008)

When comparing survivors and no survivors, the presence of lower extremity involvement or abdominal wall involvement was significantly associated with inpatient mortality

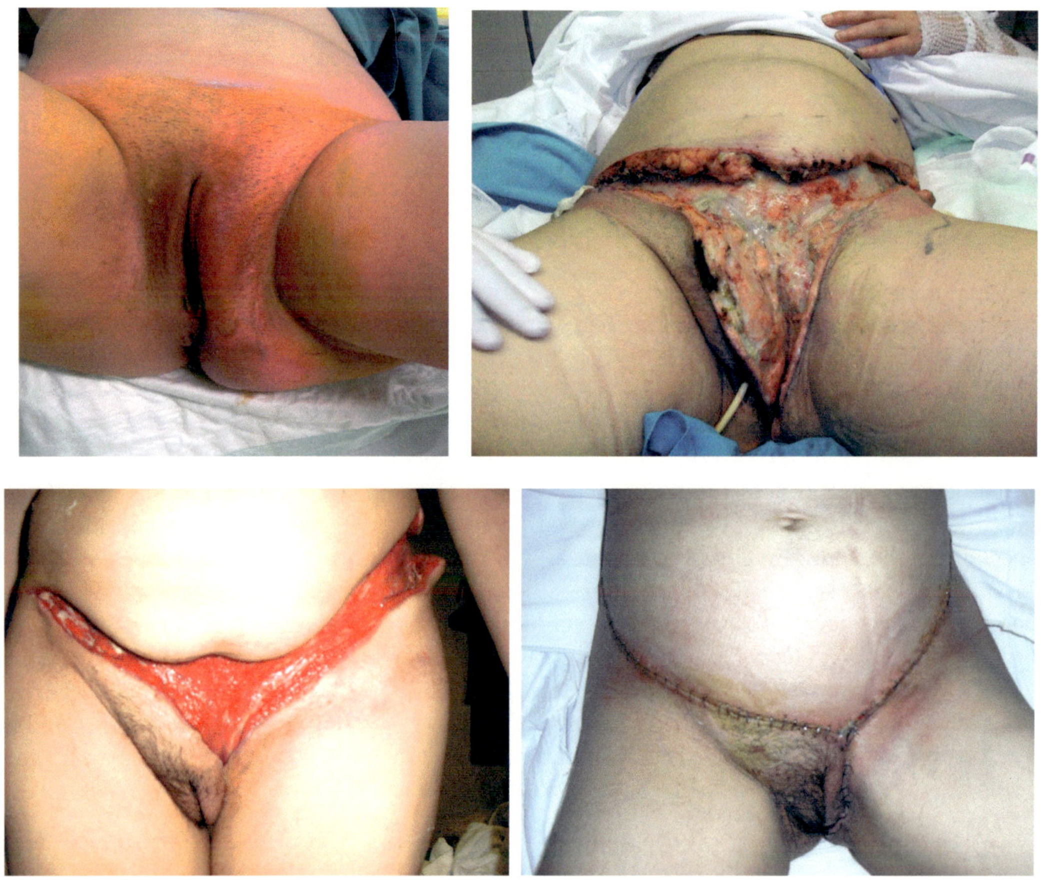

Fig. 4. Forunier's Gangrene in a young female originated in a vulvar Bartholin's abscess. See the aggressive debridement in the ilio-pubic region. In a final step a dermolipectomy was performed to close the defect. (Author's figure)

8. Annex: Proposed treatment's algorithm

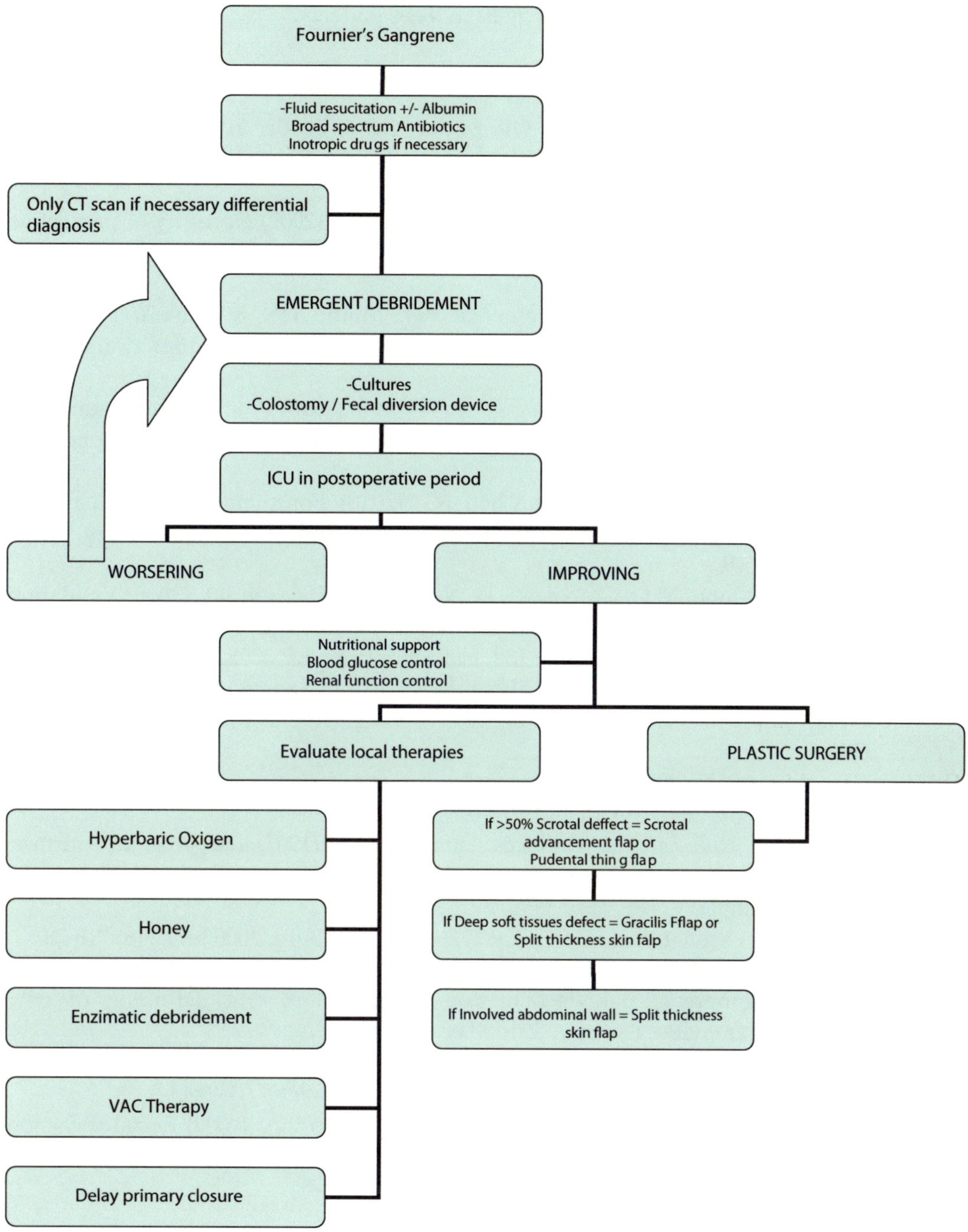

9. Conclusion

In summary, Fournier's Gangrene is a potentially fatal disease, with characteristic signs and symptoms that regularly becomes a surgical emergency. Multidisciplinary approach is essential to reduce mortality and severe sequels in these patients.

10. References

Addison WA, Livengood CH 3rd, Hill GB, Sutton GP & Fortier KJ (1984) Necrotizing fasciitis of vulvar origin in diabetic patients. Obstet Gynecol. 1984 Apr;63(4):473-9.

Akcan A, Sözüer E, Akyildiz H, Yilmaz N, Küçük C & Ok E. (2009) Necessity of preventive colostomy for Fournier's gangrene of the anorectal region. Ulus Travma Acil Cerrahi Derg. 2009 Jul;15(4):342-6.

Ameh EA, Dauda MM, Sabiu L, Mshelbwala PM, Mbibu HN & Nmadu PT. (2004) Fournier's gangrene in neonates and infants. Eur J Pediatr Surg. 2004 Dec;14(6):418-21.

Aşci R, Sarikaya S, Büyükalpelli R, Yilmaz AF & Yildiz S. (1998) Fournier's gangrene: risk assessment and enzymatic debridement with lyophilized collagenase application. Eur Urol. 1998;34(5):411-8.

Chen SY, Fu JP, Wang CH, Lee TP & Chen SG. (2010) Fournier gangrene: a review of 41 patients and strategies for reconstruction. Ann Plast Surg. 2010 Jun;64(6):765-9.

Corcoran, A.T.. Smaldone, M.C. Gibbons, E.P. Walsh T.J & Daviesb B.J. (2008) Validation of the Fournier's Gangrene Severity Index in a Large Contemporary Series. The Journal of Urology.Volume 180, Issue 3, September 2008, Pages 944-948

Corman JM, Moody JA & Aronson WJ. (1999) Fournier's gangrene in a modern surgical setting: improved survival with aggressive management. BJU Int. 1999 Jul;84(1): 85-8.

DeCastro BJ & Morey AF. (2002) Fibrin sealant for the reconstruction of fournier's gangrene sequelae. J Urol. 2002 Apr;167(4):1774-6.

De la Cruz, Alastrue, Rull, Sullana, Gratacós, Huc & Broggi (1995) Gangrena de Fournier: desbridamiento y reconstrucción en el mismo ingreso. A propósito de dos casos. Cirugía Española. Vol 59, abril 1996, número 4

Eke N. (2000) Fournier's gangrene: a review of 1726 cases. Br J Surg. 2000 Jun;87(6):718-28.

Erol B, Tuncel A, Hanci V, Tokgoz H, Yildiz A, Akduman B, Kargi E & Mungan A. (2010) Fournier's gangrene: overview of prognostic factors and definition of new prognostic parameter. Urology. 2010 May;75(5):1193-8.

Ersay A, Yilmaz G, Akgun Y & Celik Y. (2007) Factors affecting mortality of Fournier's gangrene: review of 70 patients. ANZ J Surg. 2007 Jan-Feb;77(1-2):43-8.

Estrada,O.; Martinez,I.; Del Bas,M.; Salvans S.; & Hidalgo L.A. (2009) Rectal diversion without colostomy in Fournier's gangrene Techniques in Coloproctology Volume 13, Number 2, 157-159, DOI: 10.1007/s10151-009-0474-6

Graves C, Saffle J, Morris S, Stauffer T, Edelman L. (2005) Caloric requirements in patients with necrotizing fasciitis. Burns. 2005 Feb;31(1):55-9.

Jimeno, Díaz de Brito & Parés 2010. Antibiotic tratment in Founier's Gangrene. Cirugía Española 2010;88(5):347-351

Kabay S, Yucel M, Yaylak F, Algin MC, Hacioglu A, Kabay B & Muslumanoglu AY (2008) The clinical features of Fournier's gangrene and the predictivity of the Fournier's Gangrene Severity Index on the outcomes. Int Urol Nephrol. 2008;40(4):997-1004. Epub 2008 Jun 19.

Korkut M, Içöz G, Dayangaç M, Akgün E, Yeniay L, Erdoğan O & Cal C. (2003) Outcome analysis in patients with Fournier's gangrene: report of 45 cases Dis Colon Rectum. 2003 May;46(5):649-52.

Laor E, Palmer LS, Tolia BM, Reid RE & Winter HI. (1995) Outcome prediction in patients with Fournier's gangrene. J Urol. 1995 Jul;154(1):89-92.

Laucks SS 2nd. (1994) Fournier's gangrene. Surg Clin North Am. 1994 Dec;74(6):1339-52.

Levenson RB,. Singh AK. & Novelline RA. (2008) Fournier Gangrene:Role of Imaging. Radiographics. 2008:28;520-528.

Medina Polo J, Gonzalez-Rivas Fernandez A, Blanco Álvarez M, Tejido Sánchez A.& Leiva Galvis O. (2009) Historical Review of Fournier's Gangrene: Baurienne, 1764 and Herod the Great, 4 B.C. European Urology suppl 2009; 8(4):121

Meleney FL. (1924) Hemolitic streptococcus gangrene.Arch Surg 1924

Montoya Chinchilla,R., Izquierdo Morejona,E., Nicolae Pietricicâa, B. Pellicer Francob, E., Aguayo Albasinib, J.L & Miñana Lópeza, B. (2009) Gangrena de Fournier. Análisis descriptivo de 20 casos y revisión de la bibliografía científica. Actas urol esp. 2009;33(8):873-880

Safioleas M, Stamatakos M, Mouzopoulos G, Diab A, Kontzoglou K & Papachristodoulou A. (2006) Fournier's gangrene: exists and it is still lethal. Int Urol Nephrol. 2006;38(3-4):653-7.

Sleigh, JW & Linter SPK (1985). Hazards of hydrogen peroxide. British medical journal. Volumen 291, 14 december 1985

Smith GL, Bunker CB & Dinneen MD (1998) Fournier's gangrene. Br J Urol. 1998 Mar;81(3):347-55.

Stevens DL, Bisno AL, Chambers HF, Everett ED, Dellinger P, Goldstein EJ, Gorbach SL, Hirschmann JV, Kaplan EL, Montoya JG & Wade JC; (2005)Infectious Diseases Society of America. Practice guidelines for the diagnosis and management of skin and soft-tissue infections. Clin Infect Dis. 2005 Nov 15;41(10):1373-406. Epub 2005 Oct 14.

Paty,& Smith (1992) Gangrene and Fournier's gangrene. Urologic clincics of North America 1992;19:149-62

Riseman JA, Zamboni WA, Curtis A, Graham DR, Konrad HR & Ross DS. (1990) Hyperbaric oxygen therapy for necrotizing fasciitis reduces mortality and the need for debridements. Surgery. 1990 Nov;108(5):847-50.

Yanar H, Taviloglu K, Ertekin C, Guloglu R, Zorba U, Cabioglu N & Baspinar I. (2006) Fournier's gangrene: risk factors and strategies for management. World J Surg. 2006 Sep;30(9):1750-4.

Yeniyol CO, Suelozgen T, Arslan M & Ayder AR. (2004) Fournier's gangrene: experience with 25 patients and use of Fournier's gangrene severity index score. Urology. 2004 Aug;64(2):218-22.

Part 2

Intestinal Ischemia and Bowel Gangrene

6

Intestinal Ischemia and Gangrene

Vivek Srivastava, Vaibhav Pandey and Somprakas Basu
Department of General Surgery,
Institute of Medical Sciences,
Banaras Hindu University Varanasi
India

1. Introduction

1.1 Historical background

Antonio Beniviene was the first to describe mesenteric ischemia as early as the 15th century. It was not before the mid 19th century during which the entity was extensively reported and researched after case reports by Virchow and others. The first successful surgical treatment of acute mesenteric ischmia (AMI) was performed by Elliot, who, in 1895, performed a resection of gangrenous portion of the bowel, followed by primary anastomosis of the viable parts. Dunphy correctly hypothesized that mesenteric ischemia was a manifestation of visceral atherosclerosis in the mid-twentieth century. During that time advancements in both the diagnostics and therapeutics of the disease as an entity was in full swing. Heparin was introduced for use in mesenteric venous thrombosis. In the 1950s, a major step in the vascular surgical repair to restore blood flow to ischemic bowel before gangrene occurred was introduced. The first successful embolectomy without bowel resection was performed in 1957. Nonocclusive mesenteric ischemia was first recognized as a subtype of AMI in the 1950s. By 1960, hypercoagulation status was identified as the apparent cause of most cases of mesenetric venous thrombosis and the combination of heparin administration and bowel resection became the standard treatment. In the 1970s, the use of angiography to diagnose and evaluate AMI, as well as the introduction of intra-arterial papaverine infusion, significantly improved the prognosis of patients by allowing early diagnosis and by elimination of residual arterial spasm.

1.2 Incidence

Intestinal ischemia is an uncommon condition presenting particular problems of diagnosis and management. The prevalence of the disease is difficult to establish. In the United Kingdom, approximately 2000 deaths a year are attributable to intestinal vascular insufficiency, with 1883 deaths in 2000. Of these, at least 833 (44%) were classified as acute (834 being unspecified as either acute or chronic). It affects women more than men by a ratio of 2:1. The incidence is rare below forty-five years of age and the majority of deaths occur after the seventh decade. Most cases are caused by emboli (40%-50%), followed by arterial thrombosis (25%-30%), venous thrombosis (10%), and non-occlusive mesenteric ischemia (20%). Mortality is high and has changed little since the 1970s, despite interventional advances.

2. Acute Mesenteric Ischemia

Abrupt interruption or diminution of blood flow to the intestine leads to acute mesenteric ischemia (AMI). The term AMI actually describes a wide spectrum of bowel injury ranging from reversible alterations in bowel function to transmural necrosis of the bowel wall. With better understanding of the clinical syndromes and the pathophysiological basis of AMI a multidisciplinary approach in management has emerged for patients with suspected mesenteric vascular disease. Not only is it important as a primary clinical problem causing high mortality and long-term morbidity, but also it frequently complicates other vascular conditions and operations; occurrence of colonic ischemia after aortic aneurysmectomy or aortoiliac reconstruction and the common association of superior mesenteric and peripheral arterial emboli. Acute ischemia is much more common than the chronic variant and ischemia of arterial origin is much more frequent than venous disease. AMI can result from both arterial and venous causes. The arterial forms include embolism, thrombosis, nonocclusive mesenteric ischemia and cases of focal segmental ischemia resulting from local atherosclerotic emboli or vasculitis. Acute mesenteric venous thrombosis and focal segmental ischemia caused by strangulation of the small intestine or by localized venous thrombosis comprise the venous forms of AMI.

AMI is a life-threatening vascular emergency and requires early diagnosis and intervention to adequately restore mesenteric blood flow and to prevent bowel gangrene and mortality. In spite of adequate understanding of the etiopathogenesis of the events over the past few decades, a high mortality in the range of 60%-80% associated with the disease unfortunately demonstrates a trend of continuous increase [1-5]. The main reason for this outcome is the persistent difficulty in recognizing the condition before bowel gangrene sets in [6,7].

Early clinical picture of AMI is usually nonspecific and in most cases can be characterized by an initial discrepancy between severe abdominal pain and paucity of clinical signs. Clinical examination can not differentiate an ischemic bowel from an infracted one in most cases. This is because manifestations of acute abdomen, abdominal distention and gastrointestinal bleeding may also masquerade as other abdominal emergencies. Moreover, the risk factors for AMI and the clinical course differ according to the underlying pathologic condition [8,9]. With the progression of bowel ischemia to irreversible gangrene, severe metabolic derangements ensue, leading to a series of events that culminate to multiple organ dysfunction and finally death. The timely use of diagnostic and therapeutic methods to quickly restore blood flow to the bowel is the key to reduce the high mortality associated with this condition [5,8-10].

2.1 Pathophysiology

The splanchnic circulation receives approximately 25% of the resting cardiac output, which increases by about 10% postprandial [11,12]. The mucosal and submucosal layers of the bowel receive about 75% of this blood flow. This is made possible by various factors at the cellular and the molecular level, which interact to regulate the intestinal blood flow, a mechanism that is complex and not adequately understood. The probable mechanisms include the intrinsic (metabolic and myogenic) and the extrinsic (neural and humoral) regulatory systems [12,13]. The metabolic regulatory system causes adaptive changes in splanchnic circulation depending on the amount of oxygen delivery to the tissue rather than the blood flow. An imbalance between tissue oxygen supply and demand leads to the accumulation of local metabolites (eg, hydrogen, potassium, carbon dioxide, and adenosine), which produces local vasodilatation. On the other hand, through the myogenic regulatory system, arteriolar tension receptors regulate vascular resistance in proportion to the transmural pressure. An acute decrease in perfusion pressure is compensated for by a reduction in arteriolar wall tension, thereby maintaining splanchnic blood flow. The extrinsic neural component of splanchnic blood flow regulation comprises the activation of vasoconstrictor fibers through α-adrenergic stimulation, which results in small vessel constriction and a decrease in mesenteric blood flow. Of all the types of neural stimulation (cholinergic, histaminergic, adrenergic) that affect the gut, the adrenergic limb of the autonomic nervous system is predominant. Among the humoral factors, various endogenous (epinephrine and nor-epinephrine) and exogenous factors are responsible for affecting and regulating the splanchnic circulation. Various other humoral agents, chemical mediators and cytokines like histamine, nitric oxide, leukotrienes, thromboxane analogues and glucagon can cause splanchnic vasodilatation. Pharmacologic compounds, which decrease splanchnic blood flow, are vasopressin, phenylephrine, and digoxin [14]. Dopamine, however has both vasoconstricting and vasodilating effects. In low doses it causes splanchnic vasodilation, but at higher doses causes vasoconstriction probably by stimulating α-adrenergic receptors. Other molecules like papaverine, adenosine, dobutamine, and sodium nitroprusside also increase mesenteric blood flow. Thus the splanchnic circulation is variously regulated in a complex way. Both endogenous and exogenous neuro-humoral factors, drugs and chemical mediators have significant effects on the vascular flow regulation. It is of interest that the gut tolerates hypoxia to a fair degree and the degree of reduction in blood flow that bowel can tolerate without activating these mechanisms is remarkable.

At any given time, only one-fifth of the mesenteric capillaries are open, and normal oxygen consumption can be maintained with only 20% of maximal blood flow. However, when blood flow decreases below a threshold level, oxygen consumption is reduced and oxygen debt ensues. After an attack of ischemia, when splanchnic blood flow is restored, oxygen extraction increases, providing relatively constant oxygen consumption over a wide range of blood flow rates [12]. Therefore tissue damage due to alterations in mesenteric blood flow is not only due to ischemia but more importantly as a result of cellular injury associated with reperfusion [15,16]. Mesenteric ischemia and reperfusion leads to an increase in microvascular permeability and disruption of the intestinal mucosal barrier, primarily through the actions of activated polymorphonuclear neutrophils producing reactive oxygen species and other inflammatory mediators. The tissue damage induced by the oxygen free radicals is decreased in the presence of antioxidants, xanthine oxidase inhibitors, and free-radical scavenging substances; an observation, which conclusively establishes the role of reactive oxygen species in producing cellular injury during ischemia-reperfusion [17]. In addition, phospholipase A2 is activated during reperfusion, increasing the formation of cytotoxic lysophospholipids within the ischemic tissue and up-regulating the production of prostaglandins and leukotrienes [18]. Reperfusion injury may be prevented by use of pharmacologic agents such as captopril and also carvedilol, which is an adreno-receptor blocker and a free-radical scavenger. It has also been demonstrated to have an anti-shock and endothelial-protective effect in a rat splanchnic ischemia reperfusion model [19,20].

2.2 Etiological factors

The etiology of acute mesenteric ischemia can be categorized into four specific types based on the cause of reduction of blood flow.

2.3 Arterial embolism

Emboli are the most frequent cause of AMI responsible for approximately 40% to 50% of cases [2,3]. In most situations the source of emboli is from the heart following myocardial infarction, atrial tachyarrhythmias, endocarditis, cardiomyopathies, ventricular aneurysms, and valvular disorders. These conditions can form mural thrombus, which can subsequently dislodge and embolize to the mesenteric arteries [21]. Other rare causes may include post-angiography of the coronary or cerebral circulation.

Most visceral arterial emboli lodge in the superior mesenteric artery (SMA); about 15% lodge at the SMA origin, while about 50% lodge distally at or beyond the origin of the middle colic artery [5,21]. Nearly 30% of these patients give a past history of an embolic event. The diagnosis of SMA embolism can be made intraoperatively based on the distribution of ischemia in the bowel. Since in most cases the origin the inferior pancreaticoduodenal branch is spared, perfusion of the proximal jejunum is maintained leaving the rest of the small bowel ischemic or gangrenous.

2.4 Arterial thrombosis

It is the second common cause of AMI accounting for 25% to 30% of all mesenteric ischemic events [22]. Mesenteric arterial thrombosis occurs commonly near the origin of the SMA in the setting of severe atherosclerotic disease [7]. Its slow progression allows the development of collaterals, which sustain the blood supply to a good extent. Bowel ischemia or gangrene ensues late only when the last remaining visceral artery or an important collateral artery occludes. The extent of bowel involvement is greater than that due to embolism, extending from the duodenum to the transverse colon, and results in high mortality in the range of 70% to 100% [22]. The need for more complex surgical revascularization procedures further complicates the situation.

2.5 Nonocclusive mesenteric ischemia

Non-occlusive disease accounts for about 20% of patients with mesenteric ischemia [8,23]. Its pathogenesis is poorly understood but often involves a low cardiac output state associated with diffuse mesenteric vasoconstriction possibly mediated by vasopressin and angiotensin. The mesenteric vasoconstriction commonly results from myocardial infarction, congestive heart failure, aortic insufficiency, cardiopulmonary bypass, renal or hepatic disease, major abdominal or cardiovascular surgery and vasopressor drugs [10,23]. However clear-cut risk factors may be absent. The resultant low-flow state causes intestinal ischemia and finally gangrene. It is further aggravated by endogenous and exogenous vasoconstrictors, disseminated intravascular coagulation, and cytokine-induced reperfusion injury. Both in-vitro and in-vivo studies have demonstrated the enhanced risk from the use of vasoactive drugs, particularly digoxin, in the pathogenesis of non-occlusive mesenteric ischemia (NOMI) by inducing contraction of splanchnic venous and arterial smooth muscle [14]. It has been observed that the watershed areas of circulation are more vulnerable. Patients under the stress of a surgical procedure or trauma, receiving enteral nutrition in intensive care units may also suffer from non-occlusive ischemia. The mechanism is probably due to an imbalance created between demand from the enteral feed and supply n presence of decreased mesenteric perfusion. The reported incidence of AMI in these patients is 0.3% to 8.5% and manifests with signs of sepsis, abdominal distention and ileus, which closely mimics the systemic signs of a septic state which may be already present. The mortality rate in such situations is very high, almost up to 56%, which is understandable in the context of delay in diagnosis and the already compromised state of the patient [24].

2.6 Mesenteric Venous Thrombosis

Mesenteric venous thrombosis (MVT) is the least common cause of mesenteric ischemia, representing up to 10 to 15% of all patients with mesenteric ischemia [25]. Previously they were thought of as idiopathic in nature but with the advent of improved diagnostic techniques they are now shown to be secondary to clotting disorders. [26,27]. Segmental involvement of bowel occurs starting from the venous arcades and leading to edema and hemorrhagic necrosis. This is in contrast to the thrombosis caused by the intra-abdominal causes in which the thrombus starts in larger vessels and progresses to involve the smaller venous arcades. The superior mesenteric vein is usually more commonly involved than the inferior mesenteric vein. Hence distal large bowel involvement is much less common. The transition from ischemic to normal segment is more gradual with venous occlusion than with arterial embolism or thrombosis. The mortality rate ranges from 20 to 50 percent [27] and survival depends on age, the presence or absence of co-morbid conditions, delay in diagnosis and surgical intervention. A high rate of recurrence is observed especially within 30 days of presentation [28]. A combination of surgery and anticoagulation has a lesser recurrence rate than with anticoagulation alone. The observation that most of the recurrences occur at the site of bowel anastomosis is highly significant. This reflects inadequate bowel resection or propagation of the residual thrombus, both of which indicate a gradual ischemic transition zone spread over some distance from the area of gangrene, which is vulnerable to further necrosis probably due to the propagation of thrombosis and persistent ischemia.

2.7 Clinical presentation

The signs of AMI overlap considerably with the other common acute abdominal conditions like acute pancreatitis, acute diverticulitis, small-bowel obstruction and acute cholecystitis. Moreover, the clinical features of the underlying pathology causing AMI often coexist. The patients with SMA obstruction due to embolus or thrombus have an acute onset of symptoms and a rapid deterioration in their clinical condition. This is because of the lack of collaterals leading to rapid bowel ischemia and subsequent gangrene, whereas those with NOMI or MVT have a more gradual onset and a more protracted clinical course. The hallmark of AMI is unrelenting abdominal pain. This is frequently associated with nausea, vomiting, and urgent bowel evacuation. The classic picture of a patient with acute mesenteric ischemia involves severe abdominal pain with a paucity of abdominal examination findings and a history of risk factors. Excessive fluid loss in the third space leads to mental confusion, tachycardia, tachypnea, and circulatory collapse.

Non-occlusive mesenteric ischemia occurs most frequently in the critically ill patients who have compromised hemodynamics, are often intubated and on vasopressors. They may also have coexisting severe mesenteric atherosclerosis. With an acute hemodynamic insult in the background, non-occlusive ischemia may precipitate in these patients whose mesenteric circulation is already compromised. Since they are too sick to manifest the bowel insult, delay of hours to days may occur before it is diagnosed or even suspected. A clinical clue to the problem may be an unexplained worsening in the clinical condition or a failure to thrive or a failure in having the anticipated recovery course. The typical presentation in a conscious patient not having a fulminant course is of diffuse, nonspecific abdominal pain associated with anorexia and diarrhea.

Compared with arterial thrombosis, MVT generates fewer prodromal symptoms with eating. Fever, abdominal distention, and occult blood in stool are the most common findings. Bloody ascites and large fluid losses in the third space may occur, leading to dehydration and hypotension, causing further propagation of venous thrombosis and worsening of the ischemic insult. The final outcome of all causes of mesenteric ischemia is bowel gangrene. When gangrene occurs, the patient develops peritoneal signs, hemodynamic instability, and signs of sepsis with multiorgan failure.

2.8 Diagnosis

As progression of bowel ischemia to frank gangrene is an irreversible event, prompt diagnosis and early treatment are paramount for favorable outcome in AMI. The clinician should have a high index of suspicion if the history and physical examination are suggestive of AMI [22]. Once it is suspected, prompt action to confirm the diagnosis or to exclude it should be initiated and if positive, appropriate treatment should be started without any delay. A differential diagnosis of AMI should always be kept in an elderly patient with a history of any cardiac event, like atrial fibrillation, recent myocardial infarction, congestive heart failure and arterial emboli, having postprandial abdominal pain that is out of proportion to the findings of physical examination. Survival drops rapidly from 50% when the diagnosis is made within 24 hours to 30% or less when the diagnosis is delayed [21].

The laboratory findings are nonspecific although abnormal values with clinical suspicion can help in further evaluation in line of AMI. The common laboratory abnormalities are hemoconcentration, leukocytosis, metabolic acidosis, with high anion gap and increased lactate concentrations. High levels of serum amylase, aspartate aminotransferase, lactate dehydrogenase, and creatine phosphokinase are frequently observed at presentation, but none is sufficiently specific to be diagnostic. Subacute presentation is usually seen with longer disease duration, however when ischemia from mesenteric thrombosis becomes acute, clinical presentation is similar to those who have an acute mesenteric embolic episode [29]. Hyperphosphatemia and hyperkalemia are usually late signs and are frequently associated with bowel gangrene [30]. Special laboratory tests, like serum alpha-glutathione S-transferase and intestinal fatty acid binding protein-I (I-FABP) are under evaluation [31,32].

An abdominal radiograph in AMI is also nonspecific as normal findings may be present in 25% of cases [33-35]. Characteristic radiographic abnormalities, such as thumbprinting or thickening of bowel loops, occur in less than 40% of patients at presentation. Presence of air in the portal vein is also a late finding associated with a grave prognosis [34]. The utility of a plain abdominal radiography helps to exclude other acute abdominal pathologies, such as intestinal obstruction or a perforated hollow viscus. Barium enema is contraindicated in a suspected case of AMI as increased intraluminal pressured due to barium and air can cause further reduction in perfusion, translocation of bacteria, and perforation. Moreover the presence of barium may compromise the findings of subsequent diagnostic tests, like computed tomography (CT) and angiography. Although abdominal ultrasonography is the first-line investigation for acute abdominal conditions, it is of less help in AMI even when combined with Doppler because the interpretation is often technically limited by the presence of air-filled distended bowel loops. In addition, its sensitivity is limited in detecting more distal emboli or in the assessment of NOMI. The introduction of multidetector row CT (MDCT) is a big step ahead in the evaluation of mesenteric ischemia. The use of non-ionic iodine contrast-enhanced CT scan is rapidly replacing the conventional vascular imaging techniques. MDCT and 3-dimensional imaging charecterized by high spatial resolution with a fast acquisition time provide a detailed examination of the small bowel and mesenteric vessels. The sensitivity of MDCT scan ranges from 96-100% and specificity from 89-94% [36-38]. The possible signs of mesenteric ischemia on a CT scan are thickened edematous bowel walls, hematoma, dilated bowel loops, engorged mesenteric vessels, pneumatosis, gas in mesenteric or portal veins, gangrene, and frank arterial or venous thrombosis [39,40]. Interestingly, CT is more sensitive in diagnosing MVT than other types of AMI and is considered the investigation of choice in suspected cases of MVT [41].

Selective angiography is considered to be the gold standard for the diagnosis of acute arterial occlusion with reported sensitivity ranging from 74% to 100% and a specificity of 100% [42]. Early angiography has been the major factor for the decline in mortality in patients with AMI over the past 30 years. Moreover, in the absence of mesenteric ischemia, angiography coupled with a plain abdominal radiograph may reveal the cause of abdominal pain in 25% to 40% of patients. Angiography must be bi-planar, the antero-posterior view demonstrating distal mesenteric blood supply and collaterals, and the lateral aortography for better visualizing of the origins of major visceral arteries that overlay the aorta [29]. Emboli usually lodge just after the middle colic artery where the SMA tapers. The thrombotic disease usually manifests as complete lack of visualization of the SMA origin on the lateral aortogram, associated with prominent collateral vessels in delayed antero-posterior views. Angiography also has the added advantage of being therapeutic by administration of intra-arterial thrombolytic agents for acute arterial thrombosis and intra-arterial papaverine infusion for all types of arterial ischemia. Some drawbacks of the routine use of mesenteric angiography include the technical difficulties in critically ill patients, a relatively high number of false-negatives in early course of the disease and potential renal toxicity of the contrast. Its limited availability in many centers also precludes its use as the investigation of first choice in mesenteric ischemia. MVT is characterized by a segmental slowing of arterial flow along with lack of opacification of the corresponding mesenteric or portal venous outflow tracts. In contrast NOMI has a diffuse involvement with normal venous runoff. NOMI also features a "string of sausages" sign due to multiple narrowing of the major SMA tributaries. Reflux of contrast material back into aorta is seen in venous occlusion and NOMI on selective SMA angiography.

Colonoscopy has been used to diagnose ischemic colitis but fails to visualize much of the small bowel. In addition, endoscopy may not detect subtle ischemic changes where full-blown gangrene has still not set in and these are the subset of patients who have maximum benefit from early and prompt diagnosis. Laboratory finding of elevated white blood cell counts, phosphate, lactate and lactate dehydrogenase levels in peritoneal fluid may be present in mesenteric ischemia but is usually non-specific[25,43]. Radionuclide imaging to identify infarcted bowel has been studied in animals, but clinical studies are lacking. Duplex ultrasonography has been used to detect a significant stenosis (>50%) in the mesenteric vessels in patients with chronic mesenteric arterial occlusive disease, but its role in AMI seems limited [44-47]. Although magnetic resonance imaging (MRI) has shown promise in peripheral vascular diseases but its reliability in detecting altered flows in the superior mesenteric vessels in chronic ischemia has not been documented in controlled trials [48,49]. Magnetic resonance imaging also takes longer time making its use unlikely in this rapidly progressive disorder in contrast to MDCT and angiography. Peritoneoscopy may also be a useful tool for investigating AMI due to venous thrombosis [27]. Serosanguineous fluid in the abdominal cavity of an older patient with abdominal pain, hemoconcentration, and leukocytosis is strongly suggestive of MVT. These diagnostic methods have limited use because of low negative predictive value. Clinicians must be aware that undue delay caused by insensitive and nonspecific diagnostic techniques may worsen patient outcome.

2.9 Treatment

Treatment should start as soon as the diagnosis is made. The aim is initial resuscitation, prevention of further propagation of block, prevention of reperfusion injury and early restoration of blood flow. Underlying cause, if any, should also be simultaneously treated.

Fluid resuscitation should be started early, as hydration and perfusion is important to prevent progression of clot. Ideally it should be started before angiography and should always be guided with monitoring of the central venous pressure or pulmonary capillary wedge pressure. Inotrops should be added to improve cardiac output but with precaution in NOMI, where they can aggravate bowel ischemia. Vasoconstricting agents and digitalis should be avoided if possible since they can exacerbate mesenteric ischemia. If vasopressors are required, dobutamine, low dose dopamine, or milrinone are preferred as they have lesser effect on mesenteric perfusion. Parenteral broad spectrum antibiotics should also be added to prevent bacterial translocation and sepsis. Systemic anticoagulation should be started with intravenous heparin sodium unless the patient is actively bleeding [50]. The end point of adequate heparinization is to maintain the activated partial thromboplstin time (APPT) to twice the normal value. Pain should be promptly managed, as intense pain can be a trigger for shock.

After initial supportive treatment, efforts should aim at reducing the mesenteric vasospasm. If the diagnosis of AMI is made with angiography, the angiography catheter can be used for infusion of papaverine and other vasodilators. Papaverine (30 - 60 mg/h) use is recommended in cases of arterial embolism or nonocclusive disease and has shown to improve bowel salvage by reducing vasospasm. If mesenteric angiography is not done then infusion of intravenous glucagon at 1 μg/kg per minute and titrated up to 10 μg/kg per minute as tolerated may help to reduce the associated vasospasm [50].

The main goal of treatment in patients with acute mesenteric ischemia is the restoration of intestinal blood flow as rapidly as possible. This may be achieved by medical means, endovascular procedures and by surgery. The traditional treatment of mesenteric arterial embolism has been early surgical laparotomy with catheter-based embolectomy. The appropriate therapeutic option is guided by the etiology of ischemia. A less well established approach is local infusion of thrombolytic therapy through angiographic catheter, which has been successful in a selected number of reports [51-53]. Treatment decision is guided by the presence or absence of peritoneal signs, partial or complete arterial obstruction, and on whether the location of the embolus proximal to the origin of the ileo-colic artery or in more distal branches. Thrombolytic administration is risky as bleeding is the main complication but early infusion within 8 -12 hours of onset of symptoms in the absence of peritoneal signs and distal emboli has the best outcome for successful reperfusion [54]. Surgical exploration is mandatory if clot lysis is not demonstrated within four hours or there is evidence of progressive ischemia. Long-term management is aimed at the prevention of future embolic events, typically with the use of oral anticoagulation [55].

The treatment of patients with acute mesenteric artery thrombosis is principally surgical. Surgical thrombectomy alone is unlikely to be successful in the long term. Persistence of thrombogenic atherosclerotic plaques mandates surgical thrombectomy combined with a revascularization method (arterial reconstruction, bypass or endovascular stenting). In absence of peritoneal signs with angiographic evidence of good collateral blood flow, observation while on heparin anticoagulation may be justified. The use of aspirin in the perioperative period has not been well evaluated, but it may be justified in this setting if the risk of progressive ischemia appears to be greater than the risk of bleeding. After recovery antiplatelet agents such as aspirin may reduce the risk of recurrent mesenteric ischemia [56].

The management of NOMI is essentially pharmacological and is achieved by local selective infusion of vasodilators into the superior mesenteric artery (papaverine, tolazoline, nitroglycerin, glucagon, prostaglandin E and isoproterenol) [57]. The greatest clinical experience is with papaverine administered as a continuous infusion. This approach has resulted in a reduction in mortality rates from 70%-90% to 50%-55% during the last two decades. This is followed by the patient's clinical response to vasodilator therapy from repeated angiography (ranging from 30 minutes to every 24 hours) for evaluation of vasospasm and the decision to stop papaverine infusion. Immediate laparotomy is indicated if signs of acute abdomen develop or the patient condition is worsening [58].

Standard initial treatment for acute mesenteric venous thrombosis consists of heparin anticoagulation even in patients who have gastrointestinal bleeding if the bleeding risk is considered to be outweighed by the risk of intestinal gangrene. Intra-arterial infusion of papaverine during angiography to relieve the concomitant arterial spasm is also an option. Thrombolytic therapy is still experimental and has not a clear indication in superior mesenteric vein thrombosis. Prevention of recurrent venous thrombosis with oral anticoagulation is indicated for at least six months; a longer duration may be warranted if a thrombophilic state has been identified [59].

In the presence of peritonitis or worsening of the condition on non-operative treatment, laparotomy is indicated. Fluoresceine or the Wood's lamp may help better delineation of the necrotic tissue. If a revascularization procedure is intended and resection of necrotic tissue is not imminent, it is recommended to evaluate viability after the flow restoration. After that, efforts should be made in order to minimize the reperfusion injury by administrating vasodilators and agents with free radicals neutralizing effect (allopurinol, angiotensin converting enzyme inhibitors).

A second-look laparotomy (after 24–48 hours) is recommended, even after successful primary intervention, because the intra-operative assessment of bowel viability is often inaccurate [60]. The rationale for this second look is based in part on the frequent occurrence of vasospasm after revascularization. Second-look laparoscopy has been advocated as a substitute for second-look laparotomy, but the reliability of this approach remains unproved [61, 62].

2.10 Outcome

Perioperative mortality in patients undergoing revascularization for acute mesenteric ischemia ranges from 44% to 90% [63]. Published data on long-term results after successful revascularization are few, and in general, prognosis is not as favorable as that for patients with chronic mesenteric ischemia. The most important prognostic factor is the early diagnosis. Recurrence is not uncommon, and it carries a poor prognosis. The small proportion of patients that survives massive bowel resection usually develop short-gut syndrome, requiring long-term total parenteral alimentation or small-bowel transplantation.

3. Chronic Mesenteric Ischemia

Chronic mesenteric ischemia CMI or intestinal angina is a clinical syndrome characterized by recurrent abdominal pain and weight loss due to repeated transient episodes of insufficient intestinal blood flow. This is because the increased metabolic demand falls short of the demand in the postprandial period. It occurs in the presence of severe atherosclerotic narrowing of one or more major splanchnic vessel. Approximately 90% of the patients complaining of intestinal angina have at least 2 out of 3 major mesenteric vessels occluded and 50% of them may have critical stenosis in all the 3 vessels [64]. Single vessel involvement is usually insufficient to cause intestinal angina because of the very efficient collateral circulation in the small bowel and colon. The disease is more prevalent in middle and elderly individuals with slight female preponderance in the setting of cardiovascular risk factors. The association with coronary artery, peripheral artery disease and cerebrovascular disease is seen in over 50% of patients.

3.1 Clinical presentation

The presentation of intestinal angina is due to a difference between the need of an increased blood flow required in response to food in the intestine and ability of the splanchnic circulation to meet the same. The magnitude of symptoms is dependent on the extent of atherosclerotic occlusion of the splanchnic artery. Another theory proposed is the steal phenomenon from the intestinal to the gastric circulation in response to food in the stomach [64]. Dull postprandial epigastric pain usually within the first hour after eating is the most common presentation. The intensity of pain can be of variable depending on the demand supply disparity and may occasionally radiate to the back. Heavy meals with high fat content also increase the intensity of pain. This leads to the development of a food aversion (sitophobia) and frequently, patients experience weight loss (80%). Approximately one-third of them have nausea, vomiting, and early satiety [65]. Bloating has also been observed. Constipation with fecal occult blood and ischemic colitis represent hindgut ischemia.

As with AMI the physical findings are mostly non-specific. Weight loss with signs of malnutrition, abdominal tenderness without rebound tenderness during an episode of severe pain and indirect signs of atherosclerotic vascular disease raises the suspicion of CMI. The diagnosis is mainly based on the characteristic clinical picture, the presence of an occlusive lesion in the splanchnic vessels documented by angiography and on the absence of other common causes of abdominal pain. In most cases, patients undergo an extensive workup for obscure chronic abdominal pain before the patient is seen by a vascular surgeon.

3.2 Imaging studies

A plain abdominal radiograph may suggest the diagnosis by showing calcification of the mesenteric vessels. Duplex ultrasonography of the mesenteric vessels is a useful initial test for supporting the clinical diagnosis of chronic intestinal ischemia. This should be performed by patient in fasted state because mesenteric outflow resistance changes with food intake. It is also technically difficult due to presence of bowel gas but can be accomplished in more than 85% of subjects in the elective setting. The most frequent criterion to identify the celiac artery stenosis is a peak systolic flow of 200cm/sec or more. The test has an overall accuracy of approximately 90% for detection of greater than 70% diameter stenosis or occlusion of the celiac and superior mesenteric arteries when performed in highly experienced hands [66,67]. Angiography is recommended if the results of noninvasive testing are equivocal or if they suggest that intervention is required (establishing the feasibility of revascularization) and remains the diagnostic gold standard. In order to better appreciate the lesions, acquisition must also take bi-planar views [68]. Indirect evidence of CMI may be suggested by the presence of an enlarged arch of Riolan for proximal mesenteric arterial obstruction.

Multidetector CT scans and CT-angiography allow an extensive and noninvasive evaluation of mesenteric lesions. Visualization of the collateral vessels (Riolan's arch, pancreaticoduodenal arch) and of the change in caliber of the ischemic bowel loops (stenosis) may help the diagnosis [69]. Magnetic resonance angiography (gadolinium-enhanced MRA) is highly sensitive for detecting stenosis at or near the origin of the SMA or the celiac artery and avoids the risks of radiation exposure, dye allergy and renal toxicity associated with CT scan [70]. Recent advances in MRA technology have shortened acquisition times, so it is now possible to obtain successive images in the arterial and then the portal phase. MRA can be used as an adjunct to any MR examination. Acute mesenteric ischemia is an emergency in which CT scanning is the most appropriate imaging modality. Conversely, chronic mesenteric ischemia is best examined with contrast-enhanced MRA, which is almost as accurate as digital substraction angiography [71].

Laboratory tests to evaluate malabsorption that accompny intestinal ischemia such as stool fat content, D-Xylose tolerance and Vitamin B12 absorption are non specific and generally not used in establishing the diagnosis.

3.3 Treatment

The goal of therapy for chronic mesenteric ischemia is revascularization. Taking into account the increased risk for thrombotic events with mesenteric gangrene in these patients, medical therapy alone is reserved for situation when the surgical risk is prohibitive and percutaneous revascularization is not feasible. On the other hand, medical treatment in the form of statins and antithrombotic therapy is given to all the patients except for the ones with contraindications. Oral anticoagulation may also be initiated. Analgesics and intravenous nitrates can be used for temporary pain control.

The means available for mesenteric revascularization are the surgical techniques of flow restoration and the more recently developed percutaneous transluminal procedures i.e., mesenteric angioplasty with or without stenting. As with any other vascular reconstruction patient selection and surgeon's decision combined with operative skill play an important role in overall success. The goals of these interventions are to relieve symptoms, to improve nutrition and to prevent mesenteric gangrene. Although most of the symptomatic patients have two out of three vessels involvement, the revascularization procedure should be considered in patients with documented critical stenosis in at least one major mesenteric vessel and in which other causes for chronic abdominal pain have been excluded. The indication for revascularization surgery in asymptomatic patients is not clear but it may be considered in asymptomatic patients who are submitted to aortic reconstruction for aorto-iliac occlusive disease with significant mesenteric occlusion as they have an increased risk of mesenteric gangrene after surgery [72]. Often bypass grafting of the superior mesenteric artery alone instead of complete vascularization is an effective and durable procedure for treatment of intestinal ischemia [73].

For many years, surgical revascularization has been the treatment of choice for chronic mesenteric ischemia. The techniques used include mesenteric endarterectomy and aortic reimplantation of the superior mesenteric artery. Perioperative mortality ranges from 0–11% and increases to 50% in patients with acute-on-chronic symptoms [74]. Primary graft patency rates at five years ranges from 57% to 69%, and 5-year survival rates ranges from 63% to 77% [75,76]. Postoperative morbidity rates are increased with concomitant aortic replacement, renal disease, and complete revascularization while advanced age, cardiac disease, hypertension and additional occlusive diseases influence overall mortality [77].

Percutaneous transluminal angioplasty, with or without stenting, has become an alternative to surgery for the patients, who are poor surgical candidates and for the patients in whom the diagnosis remains uncertain. The reported success rates are greater than 80% with residual stenosis of less than 50%. Relief of abdominal pain has been achieved in 75–100% patients and half of them experience weight gain. Long term follow up indicates clinical remission in approximately 80% of patients at two to three years [78]. Restenosis and recurrent symptoms occur in 17–50% of patients within the first year, making the short durability of the procedure its greatest limitation [79-83]. There has been no large randomized controlled trial comparing angioplasty, with or without stenting and surgical revascularization. As a general approach, revascularization is the treatment of choice in CMI and surgical revascularization is offered in patients with low surgical risk, while percutaneous angioplasty is preferred for high risk patients [84]. In patients who survive surgical revascularization, the prognosis is excellent and the 5-year survival rates approach 80%, with most patients becoming free of symptoms, resuming normal eating habits and gaining weight.

4. Conclusion

In summary, mesenteric ischemia is a challenging clinical problem with host of causes often diagnosed late and a strong clinical suspicion remains the key to early diagnosis. In the acute form, an aggressive approach should be adopted because the outcome crucially depends on rapid diagnosis and treatment, on the other hand, in chronic cases, the therapeutic decision should be carefully made, balancing risks and benefits, considering other comorbidities. With better understanding of the pathogenesis of mesenteric ischemia syndromes and the availability of a range of diagnostic and interventional techniques and adjuvant pharmacotherapy, an improved outcome may be achieved.

5. References

[1] Stoney RJ, Cunningham CG. Acute mesenteric ischemia. *Surgery* 1993;114:489-490.

[2] Heys SD, Brittenden J, Crofts TJ. Acute mesenteric ischaemia: the continuing difficulty in early diagnosis. *Postgrad Med J* 1993;69:48-51.

[3] Bradbury AW, Brittenden J, McBride K, Ruckley CV. Mesenteric ischaemia: a multidisciplinary approach. *Br J Surg* 1995;82:1446-1459.

[4] Lock G. Acute intestinal ischaemia. *Best Pract Res Clin Gastroenterol* 2001;15:83-98.
[5] Martinez JP, Hogan GJ, : Mesentric ischemia. *Surg Clin North Am* 2004;22:909-928.
[6] Clark ET, Gerwitz BL. Mesenteric ischemia. In: Hall JB, Schmidt GA, Wood LD, eds. Principles of Critical Care. New York, NY: McGraw-Hill Co; 1998: 1279-1286.
[7] Kaleya RN, Boley SJ. Acute mesenteric ischemia: an aggressive diagnostic and therapeutic approach: 1991 Roussel Lecture. *Can J Surg* 1992;35:613-623.
[8] Wilcox MG, Howard TJ, Plaskon LA, Unthank JL, Madura JA. Current theories of pathogenesis and treatment of nonocclusive mesenteric ischemia. *Dig Dis Sci* 1995;40:709-716.
[9] Berney T, Morales M, Broquet PE, Mentha G, Morel P. Risk factors influencing the outcome of portal and mesenteric vein thrombosis. *Hepatogastroenterology* 1998;45:2275-2281.
[10] Vicente DC, Kazmers A. Acute mesenteric ischemia. *Curr Opin Cardiol* 1999;14:453-458.
[11] McFadden DW, Rongione AJ. Intestinal circulation and vascular disorders. In: Miller TA, ed. Modern Surgical Care: Physiologic Foundation & Clinical Applications. 2nd ed. St Louis, Mo: Quality Medical Publishing; 1998:443-463.
[12] McKinsey JF, Gewertz BL, Acute mesenteric ischemia.Surg Clin North Am 1997;77:307-318.
[13] Hansen MB, Dresner LS, Wait RB. Profile of neurohumoral agents on mesenteric and intestinal blood flow in health and disease. *Physiol Res* 1998;47:307-327.
[14] Mikkelsen E, Andersson KE, Pedersen OL. Effects of digoxin on isolated human mesenteric vessels. *Acta Pharmacol Toxicol (Copenh)* 1979;45:25-31.
[15] Panes J, Pique JM, *Intestinal ischemia.* In: *Textbook of Gastroenterology*, edited by Tadataka Yamada. 5-th Edition, Blackwell Publishing, 2009, 2811–31.
[16] Zimmerman BJ, Grisham MB, Granger DN. Role of oxidants in ischemia/reperfusion-induced granulocyte infiltration. *Am J Physiol* 1990;258:G185- G190.
[17] Zimmerman BJ, Granger DN. Reperfusion-induced leukocyte infiltration: role of elastase. *Am J Physiol* 1990;259:H390-H394.
[18] Koike K, Moore EE, Moore FA, Read RA, Carl VS, Banerjee A. Gut ischemia/reperfusion produces lung injury independent of endotoxin. *Crit Care Med* 1994;22:1438-1444.
[19] Buyukgebiz O, Aktan AO, Yegen C, et al. Captopril increases endothelin serum concentrations and preserves intestinal mucosa after mesenteric ischemia-reperfusion injury. *Res Exp Med (Berl)* 1994;194:339-348.
[20] Christopher TA, Lopez BL, Yue TL, Feuerstein GZ, Ruffolo RR Jr, Ma XL. Carvedilol, a new beta-adrenoreceptor blocker, a vasodilator and free-radical scavenger, exerts an anti-shock and endothelial protective effect in rat splanchnic ischemia and reperfusion. *J Pharmacol Exp Ther* 1995; 273:64-71.
[21] Acosta S, Ogren M, Sternby NH et al. Incidence of acute thromboembolic occlusion of superior mesenteric artery-a population based study. *Eur J Vasc Endovasc Surg* 2004 ;27:145-150.
[22] Trompeter M, Brazda T, Remy CT et al. Non occlusive mesenteric ischemia: Etiology, diagnosis and interventional therapy. *Eur radiol.* 2002;12: 1179-1187.
[23] Howard TJ, Plaskon LA, Wiebke EA, Wilcox MG, Madura JA. Nonocclusive mesenteric ischemia remains a diagnostic dilemma. *Am J Surg* 1996;171:405-408.
[24] Bergan JJ, Yao JST. Chronic intestinal ischemia. In: Rutherford RB, ed. Vascular Surgery. 3rd ed. Philadelphia, Pa: WB Saunders Co; 1989:825- 842.

[25] Oldenburg AW, Lau LL, Rodenberg TJ, Edmonds HJ, BurgerCD. Acute Mesenteric Ischemia. *Arch Intern Med* 2004;164:1054-62.
[26] Abdu RA, Zakhour BJ, Dallis DJ. Mesenteric venous thrombosis: 1911 to 1984. *Surgery* 1987;101:383-388.
[27] Rhee RY, Gloviczki P, Mendonca CT, et al. Mesenteric venous thrombosis: still a lethal disease in the 1990s. *J Vasc Surg* 1994;20:688-697.
[28] Jona J, Cummins GM Jr, Head HB, Govostis MC. Recurrent primary mesenteric venous thrombosis. *JAMA* 1974;227:1033-5.
[29] Brandt LJ, Boley SJ. AGA technical review on intestinal ischemia. American Gastrointestinal Association. *Gastroenterology* 2000;118:954-68.
[30] May LD, Berenson MM. Value of serum inorganic phosphate in the diagnosis of ischemic bowel disease. *Am J Surg* 1983;146:266-268.
[31] Kanda T, Fujii H, Tani T. et al. Intestinal fatty acid-binding protein is a useful diagnostic marker for mesenteric infarction in humans. *Gastroenterology*, 1996, 110, 339.
[32] Gearhart S.L., Delaney C.P., Senagore A.J. Prospective assessment of the predictive value of alphaglutathione S-transferase for intestinal ischemia. *Am. Surg.*, 2003, 69, 324.
[33] Lund EC, Han SY, Holley HC, Berland LL. Intestinal ischemia: comparison of plain radiographic and computed tomographic findings. *Radiographics* 1988;8:1083-1108.
[34] Smerud MJ, Johnson CD, Stephens DH. Diagnosis of bowel gangrene: a comparison of plain films and CT scans in 23 cases. *AJR Am J Roentgenol* 1990;154:99-103.
[35] Wolf EL, Sprayregen S, Bakal CW. Radiology in intestinal ischemia: plain film, contrast, and other imaging studies. *Surg Clin North Am* 1992;72:107-124.
[36] Horton KM, Fishman EK. Multi-detector row CT of mesenteric ischemia: can it be done?. *Radiographics* 2001;21:1463-73.
[37] Cikrit DF, Harris VJ, Hemmer CG, Kopecky KK, Dalsing MC, Hyre CE. Comparison of spiral CT scan and arteriography for evaluation of renal and visceral arteries. *Ann Vasc Surg* 1996;10:109-16.
[38] Zeman RK, Silverman PM, Vieco PT, Costello P. CT angiography. *AJR Am J Roentgenol* 1995;165(5):1079-88.
[39] Kirkpatrick ID, Kroeker MA, Greenberg HM. Biphasic CT with mesenteric CT angiography in the evaluation of acute mesenteric ischemia: initial experience. *Radiology* 2003;229:91-98.
[40] Wiesner W. Is multidetector computerized tomography currently the primary diagnostic method of choice in diagnostic imaging of acute intestinal ischemia? [in German]. *Schweiz Rundsch Med Prax* 2003;92:1315-17.
[41] Desai SR, Cox MR, Martin CJ. Superior mesenteric vein thrombosis: computed tomography diagnosis. *ANZ J Surg* 1998;68:811-812.
[42] Grace PA, Da Costa M, Qureshi A, Sheehan S, Burke P, Bouchier-Hayes D. An aggressive approach to acute superior mesenteric arterial ischemia. *Eur J Vasc Surg* 1993;7:731-732.
[43] Kurland B, Brandt LJ, Delaney HM. Diagnostic tests for intestinal ischemia. *Surg Clin North Am* 1992; 72:85-105.
[44] Volteas N, Labropoulos N, Leon M, Kalodiki E, Chan P, Nicolaides AN. Detection of superior mesenteric and coeliac artery stenosis with colour flow duplex imaging. *Eur J Vasc Surg* 1993;7:616- 620.

[45] Harward TR, Smith S, Seeger JM. Detection of celiac axis and superior mesenteric artery occlusive disease with use of abdominal duplex scanning. *J Vasc Surg* 1993;17:738-745.
[46] Danse EM, Van Beers BE, Goffette P, Dardenne AN, Laterre PF, Pringot J. Acute intestinal ischemia due to occlusion of the superior mesenteric artery: detection with Doppler sonography. *J Ultrasound Med* 1996;15:323-326.
[47] Zwolak RM. Can duplex ultrasound replace arteriography in screening for mesenteric ischemia? *Semin Vasc Surg* 1999;12:252-260.
[48] Burkart DJ, Johnson CD, Reading CC, Ehman RL. MR measurements of mesenteric venous flow: prospective evaluation in healthy volunteers and patients with suspected chronic mesenteric ischemia. *Radiology* 1995;194:801-806.
[49] Ha HK, Rha SE, Kim AY, Auh YH. CT and MR diagnoses of intestinal ischemia. *Semin Ultrasound CT MR* 2000;21:40-55.
[50] Reinus JF, Brandt LJ, Boley SJ, Ischemic diseases of the bowel. *Gastroenterol Clin North Am* 1990;19:319-343.
[51] McBride KD, Gaines PA. Thrombolysis of a partially occluding superior mesenteric artery thromboembolus by infusion of streptokinase. *Cardiovasc Intervent Radiol* 1994;17:164-166.
[52] Rivitz SM, Geller SC, Hahn C, Waltman AC. Treatment of acute mesenteric venous thrombosis with transjugular intramesenteric urokinase infusion. *J Vasc Interv Radiol* 1995;6:219-228.
[53] Simo G, Echenagusia AJ, Camunez F, et al. Superior mesenteric arterial embolism: Local fibrinolytic treatment with urokinase. *Radiology* 1997;204:775-779.
[54] Hirsch AT, Haskal ZJ, Hertzer NR et al, ACC/AHA 2005 Practice Guidelines for the Management of Patients with Peripheral Arterial Disease. *Circulation*, 2006, 113, e463–e465.
[55] Klempnauer J, Grothues F, Bektas H, Pichlmayr R, Long-term results after surgery for acute mesenteric ischemia. *Surgery* 1997;121:239-243.
[56] Acosta S, Ogren M, Sternby NH, et al. Clinical implications for the management of acute thromboembolic occlusion of the superior mesenteric artery: autopsy findings in 213 patients. *Ann Surg* 2005;241:516-522.
[57] Kozuch PL, Brandt LJ. Review article: diagnosis and management of mesenteric ischaemia with an emphasis on pharmacotherapy. *Aliment Pharmacol Ther* 2005;21:201-215.
[58] Burns BJ, Brandt LJ. Intestinal ischemia. *Gastroenterol Clin North Am* 2003;32:1127-1143.
[59] Kumar S, Sarr MG, Kamath PS. Mesenteric venous thrombosis. *N Engl J Med* 2001;345:1683-1688.
[60] Endean ED, Barnes SL, Kwolek CJ, Minion DJ, Schwarcz TH, Mentzer RM Jr. Surgical management of thrombotic acute intestinal ischemia. *Ann Surg* 2001;233:801–808.
[61] Tola M, Portoghese A, Maniga AM. Laparoscopic second-look in acute intestinal ischemia [in Italian]. *Minerva Chir* 1997;52:527–530.
[62] Seshadri PA, Poulin EC, Mamazza J, Schlachta CM. Simplified laparoscopic approach to "secondlook" laparotomy: a review. *Surg Laparosc Endosc Percutan Tech* 1999;9:286–289.
[63] Christensen MG, Lorentzen JE, Schroeder TV. Revascularization of atherosclerotic mesenteric arteries: experience in 90 consecutive patients. *Eur J Vasc Surg* 1994;8:297–302.

[64] Paterno F, Longo WE. The etiology and pathogenesis of vascular disorders of the intestine. *Radiol Clin North Am*. Sep 2008;46(5):877-85
[65] Moawad J, Gewertz BL. Chronic mesenteric ischemia. Clinical presentation and diagnosis. *Surg Clin North Am* 1997;77:357-369.
[66] Armstrong PA. Visceral duplex scanning: evaluation before and after artery intervention for chronic mesenteric ischemia. *Perspect Vasc Surg Endovasc Ther* 2007;19:386-92; discussion 393-4.
[67] Cognet F, Ben Salem D, Dranssart M, et al. Chronic Mesenteric Ischemia: Imaging and percutaneous treatment. *Radiographics* 2002;22:863–880.
[68] Reinus JF, Brandt LJ, Boley SJ. Ischemic diseases of the bowel. *Gastroenterol Clin North Am* 1990;19:319-343.
[69] Cademartiri F, Palumbo A, Maffei E, et al. Noninvasive evaluation of the celiac trunk and superior mesenteric artery with multislice CT in patients with chronic mesenteric ischaemia. *Radiol Med* 2008;113:1135-42.
[70] Ersoy H. The role of noninvasive vascular imaging in splanchnic and mesenteric pathology. *Clin Gastroenterol Hepatol* 2009;7:270-8.
[71] Laissy JP, Trillaud H, Douek P. MR angiography: noninvasive vascular imaging of the abdomen. *Abdom Imaging* 2002;27:488-506.
[72] Thomas JH, Blake K, Pierce GE, et al. The clinical course of asymptomatic mesenteric arterial stenosis. *J Vasc Surg* 1998;27:840-844.
[73] Foley MI, Moneta GL, Abou-Zamzam AM, et al. Revascularization of the superior mesenteric artery alone for treatment of intestinal ischemia. *J Vasc Surg* 2000;32:37-47.
[74] English WP, Pearce JD, Craven TE, et al. Chronic visceral ischemia: symptom-free survival after open surgical repair. *Vasc Endovascular Surg* 2004;38:493-503.
[75] Park WM, Cherry KJ Jr, Chua HK, et al. Current results of open revascularization for chronic mesenteric ischemia: a standard for comparison. *J Vasc Surg* 2002;35:853-859.
[76] Cho JS, Carr JA, Jacobsen G, et al. Long-term outcome after mesenteric artery reconstruction: a 37-year experience. *J Vasc Surg* 2002;35:453-460.
[77] Mateo RB, O'Hara PJ, Hertzer NR, et al. Elective surgical treatment of symptomatic chronic mesenteric occlusive disease: early results and late outcomes. *J Vasc Surg* 1999;29:821–848.
[78] Florian A, Jurcut R, Lupescu I, Grasu M., Croitoru M, Ginghină C. Mesenteric Ischemia - a Complex Disease Requiring an Interdisciplinary Approach. A Review of the Current Literature. *Rom. J. Intern. Med.* 2010; 48(3): 207–222.
[79] Allen RC, Martin GH, Rees CR, et al. Mesenteric angioplasty in the treatment of chronic intestinal ischemia. *J Vasc Surg* 1996;24:415-423.
[80] Loffroy R, Steinmetz E, Guiu B, et al. Role for endovascular therapy in chronic mesenteric ischemia. *Can J Gastroenterol* 2009;23:365-73.
[81] Matsumoto AH, Tegtmeyer CJ, Fitzcharles EK, et al. Percutaneous transluminal angioplasty of visceral arterial stenoses: Results and long-term clinical follow up. *J Vasc Interv Radiol* 1995;6:165-174.
[82] Matsumoto AH, Angle JF, Spinosa DJ, et al. Percutaneous transluminal angioplasty and stenting in the treatment of chronic mesenteric ischemia: results and longterm followup. *J Am Coll Surg* 2002;194:S 22-31.
[83] Silva JA, White CJ, Collins TJ, et al. Endovascular therapy for chronic mesenteric ischemia. *J Am Coll Cardiol* 2006;47:944-950.
[84] Kasirajan K, O'Hara PJ, Gray BH, et al. Chronic mesenteric ischemia: open surgery versus percutaneous angioplasty and stenting. *J Vasc Surg* 2001;33:63-71.

Segmental Small-Bowel Gangrene Associated with *Yersinia pseudotuberculosis* Infection

H Seddik[1], A El Khattabi[2], A Abouzahir[2], O El Mansari[3],
H En-Nouali[4] and M Rabhi[5]
[1]*Department of Gastroenterology, Military Hospital, Guelmim,*
[2]*Department of Internal Medicine, Military Hospital, Guelmim,*
[3]*Department of Surgery, Military Hospital, Guelmim,*
[4]*Department of Radiology, Military Hospital, Guelmim,*
[5]*Department of Internal Medicine, Mohammed V Military Teaching Hospital, Rabat,*
Morocco

1. Introduction

Yersinia pseudotuberculosis (Y. pseudotuberculosis) is a gram- negative facultative anaerobe bacillus that can grow at low temperature (4°C). Consequently, the quantity of bacteria in food after several days of conservation in a refrigerator increases dramatically. It belongs, together with its homologue Yersinia pestis, to the family of Enterobacteriaceae. *Yersinia pseudotuberculosis* strains can be divided into 5 different *serotypes. Yersiniosis has a* wide range of clinical manifestations. The commonest is a self limiting gastroenteritis [1], but more serious variants may occur, such as appendicitis like syndrome [2] or crohn like disease [3]. We describe a small bowel necrosis associated with *Y. pseudotuberculosis* infection.

2. Case report

A 50 years old man was admitted to the emergency room with a seven day history of diffuse abdominal pain, fever, 4 time per day bloody diarrhea and weight loss. He received oral amoxicillin clavulanate two gram a day during four days without improvement. On physical examination, he had a temperature of 39 °C and a generalized abdominal tenderness to deep palpation, especially on the lower right quadrant. Laboratory work-up yielded the following: ; white blood cell count, 14.6×109 L-1; C-reactive protein,150 mg L-1 (normal <5); Renal Function, electrolytes, amylasemia, Blood and urine cultures were normal. *P*lain abdominal roentgenogram showed small bowel gas localized in the lower right quadrant. Abdominal ultrasound and CT scan showed thickening of an ileal loop and the mesenteric wall associated with intraabdominal effusion (figure 1). On the third day of admission, severe abdominal pain developed, the abdomen was protuberant, and bowel sounds were absent. Emergency exploratory laparotomy was performed. Seropurulent effusion and necrosis involving 30 cm of the distal part of the small bowel, at about 24 centimeters from the ileocecal valve was found. The mesentery appeared thickened and there was also found an extended thrombosis of all mesentery veins, draining the area of bowel necrosis. Resection of the necrotic small bowel was performed (figure 2) and histology showed extensive hemorrhagic necrosis affecting all the layers of the ileum and transmural inflammation of the ileum and the venous walls with neutrophils. Histological findings were not consistent with Crohn disease and no pathogenic organisms were cultured from the specimen. However, as suggested by histological findings, *Y. pseudotuberculosis* serology was performed and found positive with an antibody titre of 1/440, consistent with recent *Y. pseudotuberculosis* infection. Blood coagulation tests were normal. Tuberculin skin test and a Ziehl-Neelsen stain of the sputum for acid-fast bacilli, and serology for brucellosis and salmonellosis were negative. Antibiotic therapy with ciprofloxacin was started. On the twenth day post surgery the patient was discharged, in good clinical conditions.

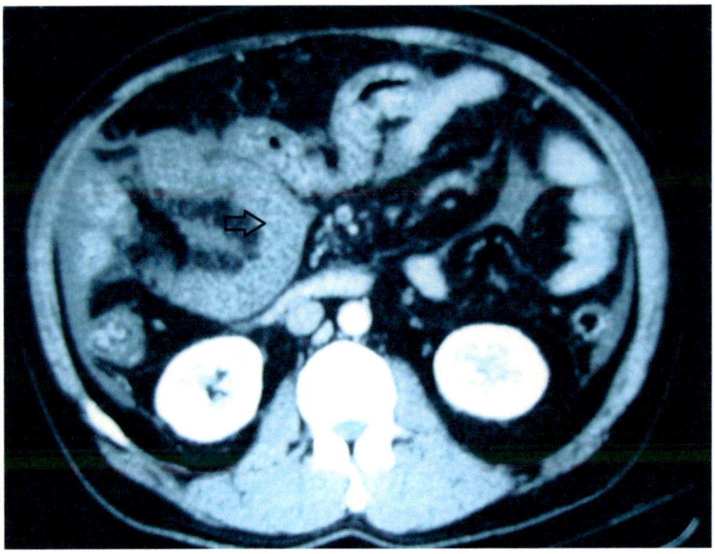

Fig. 1. Abdominal computed tomography scan with injection showing a thickened ileal loop with infiltration of its mesentery and peritoneal effusion.

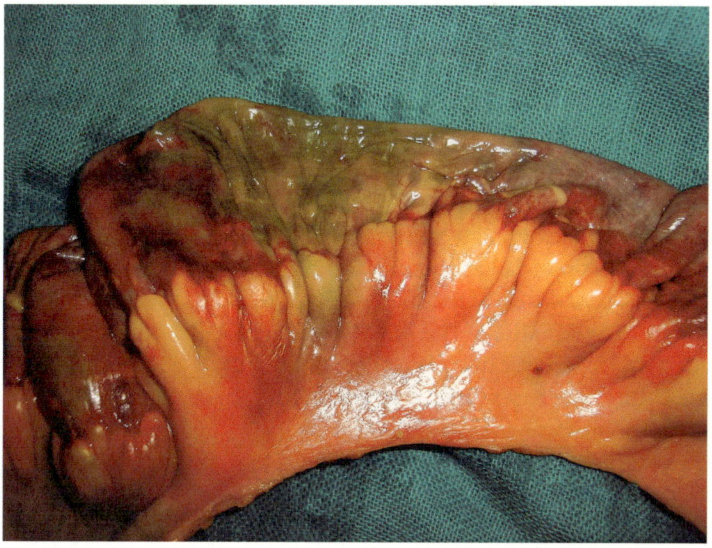

Fig. 2. Resected specimen showing necrotic ileal loop.

3. Discussion

The distribution of *Y pseudotuberculosis* infection is worldwide but it could be most commonly found in countries with cold and temperate climate. It is a bacterium isolable from the earth, from water, from a variety of foodstuffs and from human beings and animals. The animal reservoirs include many mammalian and avian hosts, such as dogs, cats, horses, cattle, rabbits, deer, rodents, and birds. An example of occupational exposure to *Y pseudotuberculosis* related to animal reservoirs involves butchers working in abattoirs slaughtering swine. *Y pseudotuberculosis* infections in humans are primarily acquired through the gastrointestinal tract after consumption of contaminated food products. Transmission may occur zoonotically, interpersonal or through consumptions of foodstuffs (in particular raw or undercooked pork products), unpasteurized milk or water not treated with chlorine. The most common manifestations of *Y. pseudotuberculosis* infection in humans are mesenteric lymphadenitis and ileocolitis accompanied by abdominal pain and fever. *Y. pseudotuberculosis* causes mesenteric lymphadenitis and may affect the appendix tissue and mimic appendicitis. Inflammation may affect the ileum and sometimes spread to the caecum simulating macroscopically Crohn's disease in its acute phase [4,5]. A mass formation, related to Y.P. infection, could occur in the right upper quadrant of the abdomen, which could be confused with tumoral lesions. Local complications due to *Y. pseudotuberculosis* have been reported rarely, such as severe bleeding, colonic perforation, subacute obstruction, and intussusceptions [6-8]. This is only one similar case of bowel necrosis following mesenteric veins thrombosis, due to *Y. enterocolitica* infection [9]. Colonic perforation and intussusception were reported in children and subacute obstruction and severe bleeding were reported in adults. We have already published a case report describing a small bowel necrosis related to *Y. pseudotuberculosis* infection [10]. Other manifestations of infection may include erythema nodosum, arthralgias, reactive arthritis, and ankylosing spondylitis. *Y pseudotuberculosis* infection has also been documented to cause lumbar facet joint disease. Acute renal failure has been reported, although very rarely. Far East scarlatinoid fever was first described in the context of *Y pseudotuberculosis* infection. A scarlatinoid-appearing rash involving the head and neck, upper and lower extremity erythema, mucous membrane enanthem, strawberry tongue and features shared with Kawasaki disease (eg, coronary artery aneurysms) characterize this syndrome. *Y pseudotuberculosis* is a gram-negative, non–lactose-fermenting coccobacillus that is chemically differentiated from other species by its fermentation of sorbitol and ornithine decarboxylase activity, among other features. The optimum growth of yersinia occurs on MacConkey medium at 20-35°C. The organism is urease-positive. Our case was negative for cultures in blood and stools, probably because of the previous antibiotic therapy. Isolation of organism from stool is difficult given the slow growth pattern and overgrowth of normal fecal flora [11]. However, stool culture yield may be increased with cold enrichment, special culture media, or alkali treatment, but these methods are generally not cost-effective [12]. Blood, peritoneal fluid, pharyngeal exudate, and synovial fluid may yield the organism. Enzyme-linked immunosorbent assay (ELISA) and agglutination tests may be obtained; the antibodies (against the O antigen) may appear soon after the onset of illness and typically wane over 2-6 months. However, cross-reaction between antibodies against other organisms may obscure the diagnostic picture. These other organisms include other *Yersinia, Vibrio, Salmonella, Brucella,* and *Rickettsia* species. Polymerase chain reaction (PCR) methods are sensitive, efficient, and accurate tools for identifying and serotyping *Y pseudotuberculosis*

[13]. Y pseudotuberculosis infection is often self-limited. However, more toxic presentations, including septic syndromes, severe dehydration, or chronic presentation, may warrant antibiotic therapy. *Yersinia enterocolitica* is susceptible to different antibiotics (aminoglycosides, tetracyclines, trimethoprin-sulfamethoxazole, ciprofloxacin) while it is in general resistant to penicillin, to ampicillin and to first-generation cephalosporin.

4. Conclusion

Yersinia may be a more important cause of acute abdominal conditions than is currently appreciated, and If specific antibody tests would have been performed routinely in every case of acute intestinal problems, the positive diagnosis of ***Y pseudotuberculosis*** could have been made much more commonly.

Conflict of interest

None

5. References

[1] Bottone EJ. *Yersinia enterocolitica:* a panoramic view of a charismatic microorganism. CRC Crit Rev Microbiol. 1977; 5: 211-41.

[2] Bottone EJ. *Yersinia enterocolitica:* The charisma continues. Ctin Microbiol Rev. 1997; 10: 257-76.

[3] Boyapalle S, Wesley IV, Hurd HS, Reddy PG. Comparison of culture, multiplex, and 5' nuclease polymerase chain reaction assays for the rapid detection of *Yersinia enterocolitica* in swine and pork products. J Food Prot. 2001 ; 64: 1352-61.

[4] Bülbüloğlu E, Ciralik H, Kantarçeken B, Cetınkaya A, Gül M, Ezbercı F. *Yersinia pseudotuberculosis* colitis presented with severe gastrointestinal bleeding. Turk J Gastroenterol. 2010; 21: 179-82.

[5] Cover TL, Aber RC. *Yersinia enterocolitica.* N Engl J Med 1989; 321: 17-24.

[6] De Berardis B, Torresini G, Brucchi M, Marinelli S, Mattucci S, Schietroma M, Vecchio L, Carlei F. *Yersinia enterocolitica* intestinal infection with ileum perforation: report of a clinical observation. Acta Biomed. 2004; 75: 77-81

[7] Grant H, Rode H, Cywes S. *Yersinia pseudotuberculosis* affecting the appendix. J Pediatr Surg 1994; 29: 1621.

[8] Leino RE, Renvall SY, Lipasti JA, Toivanen AM. Small-bowel gangrene caused by *Yersinia enterocolitica* III. Br Med J. 1980; 280: 1419.

[9] Parfenov AI, Chizhikova MD. Chronic and lingering *Yersinia* ileitis. Ter Arkh 2002; 74: 77-80.

[10] Pulvirenti D, Aikaterini T, Neri S. Septicemia, hepatic abscess, and encephalitis due to *Yersinia enterocolitica.* J Clin Gastroenterol. 2007; 41: 333-4

[11] Savin C, Carniela E. Les diarrhées d'origine bactérienne : le cas de *Yersinia enterocolitica.* Revue Francophone des Laboratoires 2008; 400: 49-58.

[12] Seddik H, Ahtil R, En-Nouali H, El Khattabi A, El Mansari O. Small-bowel gangrene revealing a *Yersinia pseudotuberculosis* infection. Gastroenterol Clin Biol. 2009; 33:118-20.

[13] Tertti R, Vuento R, Mikkola P, Granfors K, Mäkelä AL, Toivanen A. Clinical manifestations of *Yersinia pseudotuberculosis* infection in children. Eur J Clin Microbiol Infect Dis. 1989; 8: 587-91.

8

Gangrene of Large Bowel Due to Volvulus-Etiopathogenesis, Management and Outcome

Norman Oneil Machado
Sultan Qaboos University,
Oman

1. Introduction

Large bowel volvulus accounts for 10-30% of all large bowel obstruction and occurs most commonly in the sigmoid colon(Asbun 1992, Bagarani 1993, Bhatnagar 2004, Oren 2007, Pahlman 1989). It is more common in the region of Africa, South America, Middle East and Southern Asia. The most common site of volvulus include sigmoid colon(80%), caecum(15%), transverse colon(3%), splenic flexure(2%) and ileosigmoid knotting(<1%)(Bhatnagar 2004, Oren 2007, Halliday 1993, Majeski 2005, Lord 1996). Delay in presentation and diagnosis increases the risk of gangrene particularly so among the uncommon variety because of its atypical presentation and sometimes quite scarce manifestations(Bhatnagar 2004, Halliday 1993, Majeski 2005,Lord 1996). The outcome depends on intensive and adequate resuscitation with fluids and broad spectrum antibiotics and prompt resection of the gangrenous loop of gut(Asbun 1992, Bagarani 1993, Bhatnagar 2004, Halliday 1993, Majeski 2005,Lord 1996). The mortality rate even though has improved significantly in recent years due to better perioperative management of these patients, continues to remain high when gangrene sets in. The various factors that influence the outcome include general factors like advanced age of the patient, associated comorbid conditions and local factors including perforation , peritonitis and presence of shock(Bhatnagar 2004, Halliday 1993, Majeski 2005,Lord 1996, Halliday KE 1993, Feldman D 2000). This chapter intends to discuss the etiopathogenesis, presentation, investigation and management of both common and uncommon volvulus of the colon with emphasis on those volvulus being complicated with gangrene

2. Sigmoid volvulus

2.1 Introduction

Sigmoid volvulus is a leading cause of strangulation of large bowel the world over (Bhatnagar 2004, Halliday 1993, Majeski 2005,Lord 1996). It is common in Asia, Africa, Scandinavia, South America, Middle East and Eastern Europe (Bagarani 1993, Bhatnagar 2004, Oren 2007, Pahlman 1989, Halliday KE 1993, Feldman D 2000,). The incidence of gangrenous volvulus is sketchy in the world literature but the major concern is the high mortality associated with it (17 to 100%) as compared to 3-30% in non gangrenous volvulus (Bagarani 1993, Bhatnagar 2004, Oren 2007, ,Pahlman 1989). Anatomic features predisposing to sigmoid volvulus include redundant sigmoid colon that has a narrow mesenteric attachment. Sigmoid volvulus is seen in elderly patients, often in institutionalized and debilitated patients with neurological and psychiatric conditions such as Parkinson's disease and schizophrenia. The association of sigmoid volvulus with advancing age is more likely due to dysmotility rather than lengthening of the sigmoid colon and its mesentry. Other less common predisposing factors include pregnancy, post operative adhesions, internal herniations, intussusceptions, omphalomesenteric abnormalities, intestinal malrotation, appendicitis and carcinoma. (Bhatnagar 2004, Oren 2007, Pahlman 1989, Halliday KE 1993, Feldman D 2000)

2.2 Presentation

The predominant symptom of gangrenous sigmoid volvulus is abdominal pain and progressive abdominal distension (92 to 95%), constipation (92%), muscle guarding / rigidity (75%) and vomiting in 60% of the cases (Asbun 1992, Bagarani 1993, Bhatnagar 2004, Oren 2007, Pahlman 1989). A visible sigmoid loop is noted in 42% and rectal examination may reveal blood in the examination finger. The median duration of symptom on admission is 3 days (3.7±2.8 range 1-15) (Asbun 1992, Bagarani 1993, Bhatnagar 2004, Oren 2007, ,Pahlman 1989). A previous attack of volvulus is recorded in 23.5% while 72.5% may develop gangrene in the first attack (Bhatnagar 2004). The incidence of preoperative shock did not differ in patients with differing pattern of gangrene but the incidence of shock is significantly higher in patient who died (Bagarani 1993, Bhatnagar 2004, Oren 2007, ,Pahlman 1989, Halliday KE 1993).

2.3 Pattern of gangrene

Gangrene of the colon may be extensive and well defined (figure 1) or at times may be patchy with ill defined limits. The pattern of gangrene can be divided into 3 groups (Bhatnagar 2004): (a) those with gangrene confined to sigmoid colon. In 73% of the cases the gangrene is confined classically to the area of constriction. (b) the gangrenous area may extend beyond the confines of the area under constriction on one or both sides (26% of the cases)(Bhatnagar 2004). More often it extends well down into the rectum lying in the hallow

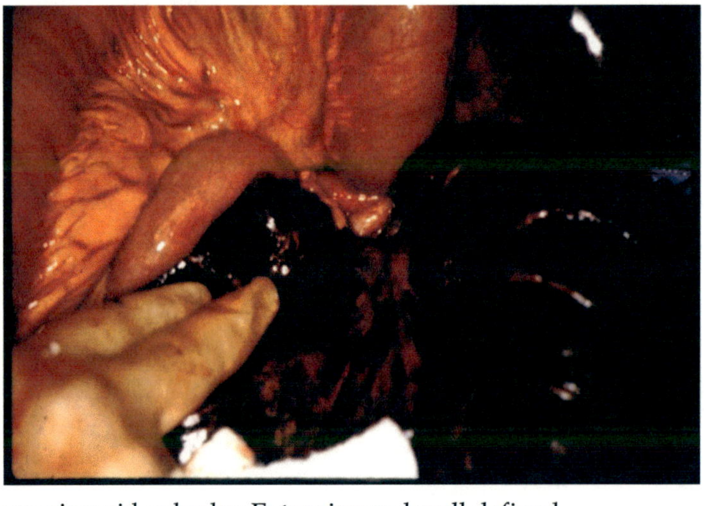

Fig. 1. Gangrenous sigmoid volvulus-Extensive and well defined

of the sacrum(c) those with gangrene of the sigmoid with ileal knotting. In 15%, the gangrenous sigmoid may be involved in knotting with ileum. The gangrene of rectum distal to the twist is uncommon as the main vascular supply to the rectum lies proximally running in the medial limb of the sigmoid mesocolon and hence is generally not involved in the twist. However it could be involved if the vessels take a slightly aberrant lateral course in the mesocolon which is narrowed and hence can become incorporated in the twist. If the gangrene in rectum distal to the twist is not recognized, it can lead to an error in judgment of performing an anastomosis to the gut of questionable viability and with disastrous consequences (Asbun 1992, Bhatnagar 2004)

2.4 Investigations

The diagnosis could be established in approximately 60% of the cases with a plain x-ray abdomen (Bhatnagar 2004, Oren 2007, ,Pahlman 1989, Halliday KE 1993, Feldman D 2000). The distended sigmoid colon appears as ahaustral collection of gas (sometimes referred as "bent inner tube" sign or "coffee bean" sign) that extends from the pelvis to the right upper quadrant as high as the diaphragm(Feldman D 2000). Distended large bowel proximal to the sigmoid colon and air fluid levels in the small bowel are often present (Asbun 1992, Bagarani 1993, Bhatnagar 2004, Oren 2007, Pahlman 1989, Ballantyne GH 1982). Presence of air in the bowel wall (pneumatosis intestinalis), free air in peritoneal cavity or in the portal vein would strongly indicate the presence of gangrenous gut. A barium enema with water soluble contrast is contraindicated when gangrene is suspected(Mellor MF 1994) . A CT scan would show the typical finding of a whirl sign at the site of the twist caused by dilated sigmoid colon around its mesocolon and vessels and bird beak appearance of the afferent and efferent colonic segment (Catalano O 1996).

2.5 Management

It is of outmost importance to be aware that a gangrenous volvulus is an acute surgical emergency and has to be dealt expeditiously and aggressively to achieve better outcome. The management of sigmoid volvulus involves adequate and prompt fluid resuscitation, decompression of proximal bowel and urgent resection of the gangrenous segment (Asbun 1992, Bagarani 1993, Bhatnagar 2004, Oren 2007, Pahlman 1989, Ballantyne GH 1982, Kuzu MA 2002) . While in the absence mucosal ischemia it would seem reasonable to attempt detorsion and decompression via sigmoidoscopic placement of soft rectal tube or occasionally barium enema(Mellor MF 1994), the presence of gangrene of colon warrants immediate laparotomy after intensive resuscitation(Bhatnagar 2004, Ballantyne GH 1982, Kuzu MA 2002). In gangrenous sigmoid volvulus, resection and primary anastomosis may be performed with acceptable mortality and morbidity rates provided that the patients is haemodynamically stable and a tension free anastomosis of well vascularised segments of the bowel is feasible. This technique when employed has a reported mortality rate of 16 to 33%(Oren 2007, ,Pahlman 1989,Bhatnagar 2004, Ballantyne GH 1982, Kuzu MA 2002) .On table cleaning of the proximal bowel may be added to perform the primary anastomosis with reasonable safety. When condition for primary anastomosis is not ideal then Hartmann's operation or Mickulicz procedure with resection of gangrenous loop may be life saving particularly in unstable patients with severe fecal peritonitis((Bhatnagar 2004, Kuzu MA 2002). The drawback of adding a stoma however is that it carries the mortality and morbidity risks associated with stoma and that it requires a second operation.

2.6 Outcome

The mortality following surgery in these patients range from 19 to 66%(Asbun 1992, Bagarani 1993, Bhatnagar 2004, Oren 2007, ,Pahlman 1989, Ballantyne GH 1982, Kuzu MA 2002) . Experienced surgeons however could perform both primary anastomosis and stoma successfully by laparoscopic approach; the concern however is that of rupture of gangrenous loop while doing so. Exteriorisation of the gangrenous gut is another option although it is difficult to fully exteriorize a gangrenous loop and the associated mortality could be higher(Asbun 1992, Bagarani 1993, Bhatnagar 2004, Oren 2007, ,Pahlman 1989, Ballantyne GH 1982, Kuzu MA 2002). While the overall mortality in nongangrenous sigmoid volvulus is 6 to 24%, in gangrenous SV it ranges from 11 to 80% (Asbun 1992, Bagarani 1993, Bhatnagar 2004, Oren 2007, Pahlman 1989, Kuzu MA 2002). The factors that influence the adverse outcome include delay in presentation or diagnosis, advanced age, fecal peritonitis due to perforation of gangrenous loop, previous episodes of volvulus, associated comorbidities including diabetes mellitus, and renal, cardiac and pulmonary insufficiency (Asbun 1992, Bagarani 1993, Bhatnagar 2004, Oren 2007, Pahlman 1989, Ballantyne GH 1982, Kuzu MA 2002). The most important cause of death however is septicaemic shock. The morbidity rate is approximately 6 to 26% and includes wound infection, intra-abdominal abscess, evisceration, anastomotic leakage, stomal complications, intestinal obstruction, respiratory complications and DVT(Asbun 1992, Bagarani 1993, Bhatnagar 2004, Oren 2007, ,Pahlman 1989). The mean hospitalization period ranges from 8 to 13 days (Bhatnagar 2004). Since gangrenous SV invariably requires resection of sigmoid colon, recurrence of volvulus is unlikely (Asbun 1992, Bagarani 1993, Bhatnagar 2004, Oren 2007, Pahlman 1989).

2.7 Summary

Gangrenous sigmoid volvulus invariably occurs due to delay in presentation or diagnosis. The occurrence of gangrene beyond the confines of twist is likely and awareness of this is necessary to avoid insecure anastomosis. The management includes aggressive resuscitation followed by resection of the gangrenous loop with primary anastomosis or stoma. The mortality is significantly higher than in patients with nongangrenous sigmoid volvulus. Various factors that would influence the outcome adversely is older age group, associated comorbidities, presence of shock at admission, fecal peritonitis and previous episode of volvulus.

3. Cecal volvulus

3.1 Introduction

Cecal volvulus (CV) is an axial twist of the cecum ascending colon and terminal ileum around a mesenteric pedicle. CV is relatively uncommon with an incidence of 2.8 to 7.1 per million people per year(Tejler G 1988).Cecal volvulus occurs in patients who have increased cecal motility as a result of anomalous fixation of the right colon. Acquired anatomical abnormalities such as surgical adhesions can also contribute. Other conditions that have been associated with cecal volvulus include pregnancy, congenital malformations, colonoscopy, Hirschprung's disease and mobile cecal syndrome(Tejler G 1988, Bystrom J 1972, Madiba TE 2002). The majority of the patients with cecal volvulus have full axial rotation causing twisting of the mesentery and blood vessels (Majeski J 2005, Tejler G 1988, Bystrom J 1972). In approximately 10% of cases the cecum and ascending colon fold in the anterior cephalad direction (known as cecal bascule)(Tejler G 1988, Bystrom J 1972).

Although cecal bascule does not cause torsion of the mesentery and blood vessels it can lead to intestinal gangrene due to distension and bowel wall ischemia(Tejler G 1988, Bystrom J 1972).

3.2 Presentation

The majority of patients with cecal volvulus have similar presentation to those with small bowel obstruction (Majeski J 2005, Tejler G 1988, Bystrom J 1972, Madiba TE 2002). The major symptoms are abdominal pain, nausea, vomiting and obstipation. The pain is usually steady with superimposed colicky component associated with peristalsis. The abdomen is often diffusely distended representing the dilated right colon and small bowel. Fever, peritonitis or hypotension may indicate the presence of intestinal gangrene (Majeski J 2005, Tejler G 1988, Bystrom J 1972, Madiba TE 2002).

3.3 Investigations

The diagnosis can be established by a barium or water soluble contrast enema or CT scan(Majeski J 2005, Tejler G 1988, Bystrom J 1972, Madiba TE 2002). On plain radiography the cecum appears as a kidney shaped mass extending into the left upper quadrant. Distended loop of small bowel are common. The abdominal plain film is suggestive of diagnosis in 46% but diagnostic only in 17% of the cases(Majeski J 2005, Tejler G 1988, Bystrom J 1972). While barium study is diagnostic in 88% of the cases it is contraindicated when diagnosis is not clear or gangrene is suspected (Tejler G 1988, Bystrom J 1972). CT scan has become the preferred radiological test for establishing the diagnosis of cecal volvulus and in recognizing its variant. It can also show the signs of strangulation and or perforation (Tejler G 1988, Bystrom J 1972).

3.4 Management

While the goal of nongangrenous cecal volvulus is to prevent the development of gangrene and address the anatomic abnormality, in gangrenous volvulus the need of the hour is resection of gangrenous loop immediately after adequate resuscitation (Majeski J 2005, Tejler G 1988, Bystrom J 1972, Madiba TE 2002). While several techniques may be used in dealing with nongangrenous cecal volvulus including cecopexy and cecostomy, in the presence of gangrene the surgical approach warrants resection of gangrenous gut and primary anastomosis (Madiba TE 2002). Colopexy of the remainder right colon would be required as in most instances the right colon is mobile due to failure of fusion of the cecum and ascending colon to posterior pericolic peritoneum(Madiba TE 2002). The tinea of reminder of the right colon holds sutures very well because this segment of the colon is not involved in cecal volvulus. The remainder of the distal colon must always be carefully examined intra-operatively for colonic obstruction. A proximal ileocolic anastomosis in the presence of a distal obstruction may lead to a lethal postoperative outcome (Majeski J 2005, Madiba TE 2002).

3.5 Outcome

The outcome of resection of gangrenous cecal volvulus depends on the overall fitness of the patient including the age and associated comorbid conditions. The overall mortality in gangrenous cecal volvulus range from 23 to 48% (Majeski J 2005, Tejler G 1988, Bystrom J 1972, Madiba TE 2002). The presence of preoperative shock and fecal peritonitis have adverse outcome.

4. Splenic flexure volvulus

4.1 Introduction

The splenic flexure volvulus is rare with an incidence of less than 2% of all colonic volvulus with approximately 32 cases being reported in the literature so far(Ballantyne GH 1985). The rarity of the splenic flexure volvulus is due to the fact that this part of large bowel has limited mobility due to its attachment to phrenocolic, gastrocolic and splenocolic ligament and intraperitoneal position of the descending colon(Ballantyne GH 1985,Mittal R 2007, Osuka A 2006). For splenic flexure volvulus to occur some or all of these anatomical factors should be congenitally absent or altered by surgery thus rendering the flexure unusually mobile. The splenic flexure volvulus has also been reported with other congenital anomalies including wandering spleen causing volvulus of the splenic flexure; this causes partial obstruction of the large intestine by the splenic pedicle(Ballantyne GH 1985,Mittal R 2007). Congenital bands and acquired adhesions due to previous surgeries could be other etiological factors (Ballantyne GH 1985, Mittal R 2007, Osuka A 2006) .

4.2 Presentation

Though there are reported cases of splenic flexure volvulus in children(Osuka A 2006) the median age of these patients is 53 years with a female preponderance (Ballantyne GH 1985, Mittal R 2007). The usual presentation of these patients is non acute and nonspecific and include recurrent episodes of abdominal pain, distension and vomiting and is usually not suspected because of the rarity of this condition. Acute presentation with features of gangrene is rare (figure 2) and such patients could present with severe tenderness, guarding, rigidity and shock invariably due to delay in presentation or diagnosis (Ballantyne GH 1985, Mittal R 2007, Osuka A 2006).

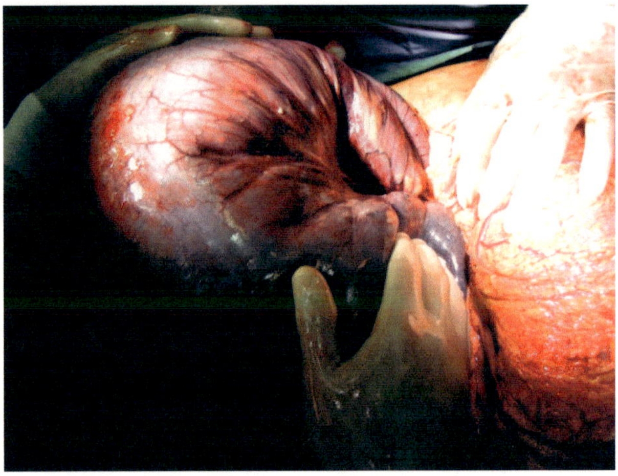

Fig. 2. Splenic flexure volvulus- grossly distended gangrenous loop

4.3 Investigations

Diagnosis of this rare condition is facilitated by radiological investigation including plain X-ray abdomen and CT scan(Ballantyne GH 1985,Mittal R 2007, Osuka A 2006). The characteristic findings include the following: 1) two widely separated air fluid levels one in the distended splenic flexure and the other in the cecum (figure 3); 2)markedly dilated air filled colon with abrupt termination at the anatomic splenic flexure; 3)an empty descending and sigmoid colon; 4) a characteristic beak at the anatomic splenic flexure on barium enema examination if performed; 5) a coffee bean appearance of the dilated splenic flexure is seen

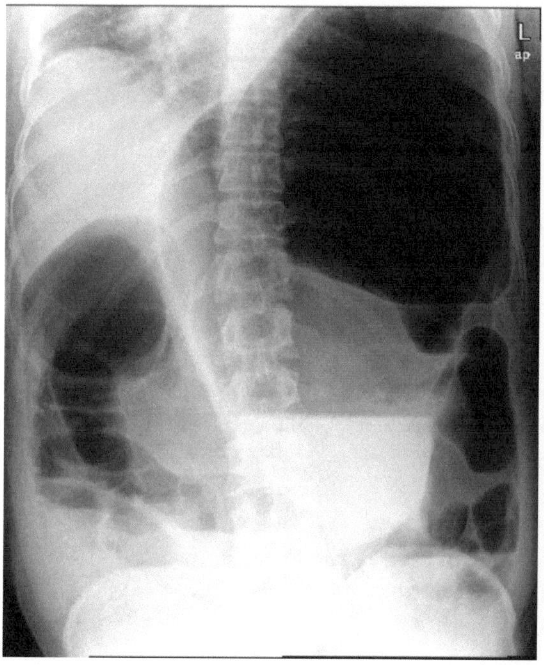

Fig. 3. Plain x-ray showing two widely separated air fluid levels in splenic flexure and cecum

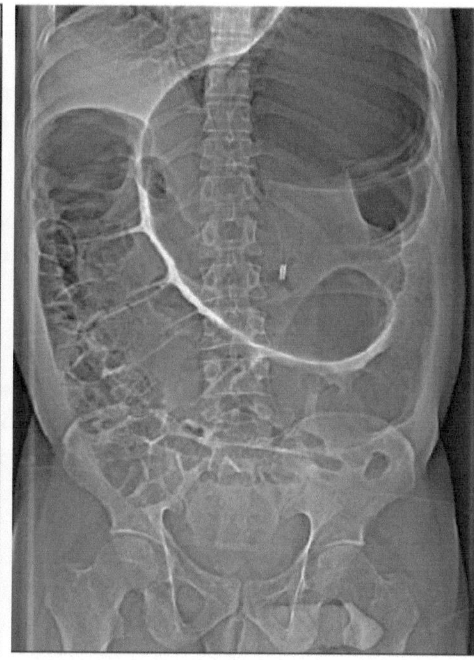

Fig. 4. CT scout film revealing dilated splenic flexure loop with concavity facing upwards and laterally

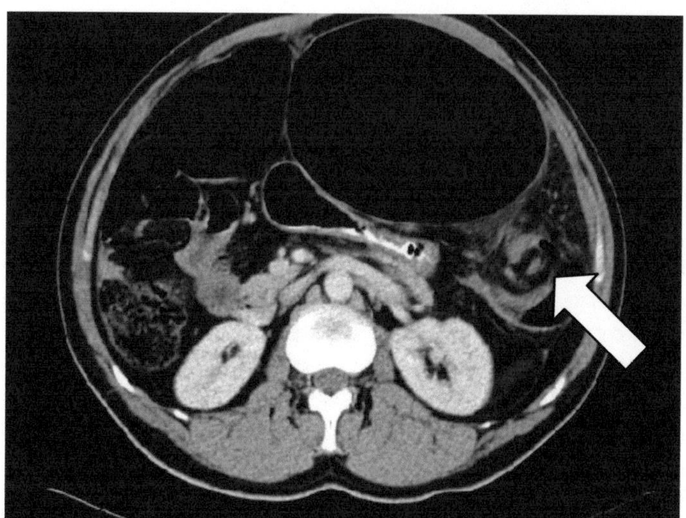

Fig. 5. CT image showing dilated splenic flexure with whirl sign (arrow)

and in splenic flexure volvulus unlike sigmoid volvulus the concavity of the bean is facing upwards and laterally (figure4). The CT scan will reveal dilated splenic flexure with a characteristic whirl sign at the site of the twist of the mesentery[6] (figure 5). The presence of gangrene is suspected when there is air in the wall of the bowel (pneumatosis intestinalis), air in portal vein or in the presence of peritonitis[6].

4.4 Management

Like in the case of sigmoid volvulus the immediate priority is aggressive resuscitation with IV fluids and appropriate antibiotics to optimize the patient for an urgent surgery (Ballantyne GH 1985, Mittal R 2007, Osuka A 2006). The broad principle of management would include resection and primary anastomosis or creation of stoma. A primary anastomosis is avoided in the presence of perforation and peritoneal soiling, preoperative shock and in the presence of dilated edematous loops of gut to be anastomosed (Ballantyne GH 1985, Mittal R 2007, Osuka A 2006).

4.5 Outcome

The overall mortality ranges from 16 to 33% and depends significantly in delay in diagnosis, presence of shock, fecal peritonitis and associated comorbidities (Ballantyne GH 1985, Mittal R 2007, Osuka A 2006).

4.6 Summary

Splenic flexure volvulus is a rare cause of intestinal obstruction. Gangrene is usually associated with the acute form of presentation. Rarity of the condition and protean manifestation may lead to delay in the diagnosis. Radiological investigations could however guide to a prompt surgical treatment after adequate resuscitation. Resection and primary anastomosis is often feasible failing which the patient my require resection with colostomy.

As the manifestation of transverse colon volvulus is to a large extent similar to splenic flexure volvulus it would not be further discussed.

5. Ileosigmoid knotting

5.1 Introduction

Ileosigmoid knotting is a rare cause of intestinal obstruction that rapidly progresses to gangrene of ileum as well as the sigmoid colon(Shepherd JJ 1967,Puthu D 1991, Alver O 1993). Preoperative diagnosis is difficult because of its infrequency and atypical radiographic findings (Shepherd JJ 1967). It is essential to differentiate it from sigmoid volvulus because endoscopic reduction is a contraindication in ISK(Raveenthiran V 2001). In recent years CT has been useful in making a preoperative diagnosis (Raveenthiran V 2001). Generalized peritonitis and sepsis are the main cause of poor outcome (Shepherd JJ 1967, Puthu D 1991, Alver O 1993). After hemodynamic stabilization, immediate surgical intervention is need of the hour. Three factors are responsible for ileosigmoid knotting (Shepherd JJ 1967): 1) a long small bowel mesentery and freely mobile small bowel 2) a long sigmoid colon on a narrow pedicle and 3) ingestion of high bulk diet in the presence of empty small bowel as would happen during the fasting month of Ramadan among Muslims. When a semi liquid bulk meal progresses into the proximal jejunum it increases the mobility of the intestine and the heavier segments of the proximal jejunum fall into the left lower quadrant(Shepherd JJ 1967). The empty loop of ileum and distal jejunum twist in a clockwise rotation around the base of the narrow sigmoid colon. Further peristalsis form an ileosigmoid knot with 2 closed loop obstruction; one in the small bowel and the other in the sigmoid colon. Ileo sigmoid knotting is categorized into 3 types (Shepherd JJ 1967). In type 1, the ileum (active component) wraps itself around the sigmoid colon (passive component) in a clockwise or anticlockwise direction. In type 2 the sigmoid colon (active component) wraps itself around a loop of ileum (passive component) in a clockwise or anticlockwise direction and in type3 the ileocecal segment (active component) wraps itself around the sigmoid colon (passive component)

5.2 Presentation

Ileosigmoid knot rapidly progresses to gangrene of ileum as well as the sigmoid colon. (Figure 6). Generalized peritonitis ,sepsis and dehydration are the principal complications (Shepherd JJ 1967, Puthu D 1991, Alver O 1993, Raveenthiran V 2001). The predominant symptom and signs of presentation include abdominal pain and tenderness (100%), abdominal distension (94 to 100%), nausea and vomiting (87 to 100%), rebound tenderness (69%) and shock (0 to 60%)(Shepherd JJ 1967, Puthu D 1991, Alver O 1993, Raveenthiran V 2001). Despite the critical condition the preoperative diagnosis is not easy. The diagnostic difficulty is partly caused by the unfamiliarity of this rare entity and the confusing and self contradicting feature of the disease. While the clinical feature of vomiting suggests small bowel obstruction the radiographic findings are that of colonic distension which is uncommon in small bowel obstruction. In 73 to 79.5% of cases the bowel is gangrenous (Shepherd JJ 1967,Puthu D 1991, Alver O 1993, Raveenthiran V 2001). Both sigmoid colon and small bowel are involved in 52 to 60% of the cases. Paradoxically the incidence of bowel gangrene was 90% in those who presented early within 24 hours of their symptoms, presumably reflecting the fulminating clinical deterioration of patients due to early and extensive infarction of the bowel involved in a tight knot(Horgan PG 1992). In patients who present after 24 hours of the initial symptoms the bowel gangrene was noted in 57% of the cases.(Shepherd JJ 1967, Puthu D 1991, Alver O 1993, Raveenthiran V 2001).

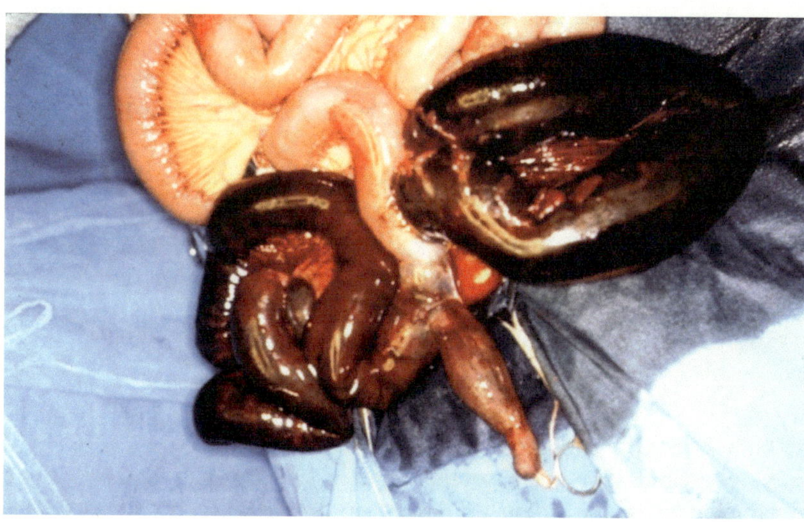

Fig. 6. Ileosigmoid knot- Gangrenous ileum and sigmoid colon seen along with the Meckel's diverticulum

5.3 Investigations

The diagnosis could be achieved following radiological investigations. The plain X-ray findings include a double loop of dilated sigmoid colon and multiple air fluid levels in the small intestine(Shepherd JJ 1967,Puthu D 1991, Alver O 1993, Raveenthiran V 2001)). The CT scan findings suggestive of Ileo sigmoid knot include the whirl sign created by the twisted intestine and sigmoid mesocolon in the ileosigmoid knot, medial deviation of cecum and ascending colon (Alver O 1993, Raveenthiran V 2001).

5.4 Management

The initial management would involve aggressive resuscitation with fluid, appropriate antibiotics and correction of acid base imbalance if any (Shepherd JJ 1967,Puthu D 1991, Alver O 1993, Raveenthiran V 2001). After hemodynamic stabilization, laparotomy is performed without any delay. The outcome would depend significantly in early and adequate resuscitation and prompt resection of the gangrenous loop. Various surgical procedures have been employed in these patients. The initial attempt to untie the knot may be feasible when both sigmoid and ileum are viable or sigmoid colon alone is viable (Shepherd JJ 1967, Puthu D 1991, Alver O 1993, Raveenthiran V 2001). When both sigmoid and ileum are gangrenous there is difficulty in untying the knot with the potential risk of rupture of the gangrenous loop in doing so leading to peritoneal spillage of the toxic bowel contents (Shepherd JJ 1967,Puthu D 1991, Alver O 1993, Raveenthiran V 2001). Intestinal clamps hence should be applied before dissection or resection of the knot and the loops.

Primary anastomosis of the small bowel loop after resection is preferable(Raveenthiran V 2001). When the terminal ileum is gangrenous within 10 cms of the ileocecal valve an end to end anastomosis is avoided(Raveenthiran V 2001). The distal stump is then closed and end to side ileocecostomy is performed. Resection of the sigmoid colon is often advised even when it is viable to prevent recurrent volvulus and recurrent knotting(, Alver O 1993, Raveenthiran V 2001). Primary anastomosis following colonic resection could be carried out safely particularly when the history is short and the remaining bowel is clean, well vascularalised and undistended and a tension free anastomosis is feasible. In the absence of an ideal situation and significant preoperative shock or peritoneal contamination a Hartmann procedure or covering colostomy may be advocated to avoid the risk of fecal leak from colonic anastomosis (Shepherd JJ 1967,Puthu D 1991, Alver O 1993, Raveenthiran V 2001).

5.5 Outcome

The operative mortality from ileo sigmoid knot varies from 0 to 48% (mean 35.5%). The mortality figures are generally related to duration of the symptom, preoperative shock, the presence or absence of gangrene and the general status of the patient(Shepherd JJ 1967,Puthu D 1991, Alver O 1993, Raveenthiran V 2001).

5.6 Summary

Ileo sigmoid knot is a rare cause of intestinal obstruction. Unfamiliarity and diagnostic difficulties have contributed to the mortality and morbidity of this condition in the past. Better understanding of the problem and increased possibility of preoperative diagnosis following CT scan have facilitated early diagnosis and intervention. Aggressive fluid resuscitation, preoperative antibiotics, prompt laparotomy and effective surgery including resection of gangrenous loop and primary anastomosis and better perioperative care of the shocked patient have optimized the survival of these patients

6. General considerations in management of ischemic gut

While an obviously gangrenous bowel is easy to detect, operative evaluation to determine the viability of borderline ischemia may not be precise(Horgan PG 1992). The use of intraoperative doppler examination and use of intravenous administration of fluroscein with visual examination using ultraviolet light are standard methods to determine bowel viability(Horgan PG 1992). These intraoperative tests are not absolutely accurate. Moreover both tests require detorsion of the bowel and reperfusion of the bowel. Reperfusion of ischemic or gangrenous bowel can produce metabolic acidosis, intestinal bacterial and toxin translocation and possible irreversible septic shock(Patel A 1992, Zimmerman BJ 1992). Reperfusion of ischemic intestine results in extensive microvascular and parenchymal cell injury by release of proteases and physical disruption of the endothelial barrier resulting in eventual cell death(Zimmerman BJ 1992). To avoid reperfusion of the ischemic volvulus and reperfusion injury the gangrenous bowel loop should be resected without detorsion (Alver O 1993, Raveenthiran V 2001)

7. Summary

Gangrene is a potential complication of colonic volvulus. It is of outmost importance that a clinician avoids this complication in a patient with a colonic volvulus by an early diagnosis, adequate resuscitation and prompt surgical intervention. Once gangrene has set in the outcome is adversely effected. The surgical intervention would involve resection with primary anastomosis or creation of stoma. Primary anastomosis is generally avoided in the presence of shock, significant peritonitis, and inability to create anastomosis between two well vascularised loops in a tension free manner. The factors that seriously affect the outcome include general factors including advanced age and associated comorbid conditions and local factors including fecal peritonitis and shock

8. References

[1] Alver O, Oren D, Tireli M, Kayabasi B, Akdemir D, ileosigmoid knotting in turkey: review of 68 cases. Dis Colon Rectum.1993;36(12):1139-47

[2] Asbun HJ, Castellenos H, Balderrama B, Ochoa J, Arismendi R, Teran H, Asbum J. sigmoid volvulus in the high altitude of the Andes- review of 230 cases. Dis Colon Rectum.1992;35(4) :350-3

[3] Bagarani M, Conde AS, Longo R, Italiano A, Terenzi A, Venuto G. Sigmoid volvulus in West Africa: a prospective study on surgical treatments. Dis Colon Rectum. 1993;36:186-90

[4] Ballantyne GH. Review of sigmoid volvulus: history and results of treatment. Dis colon Rectum.1982;25(5):494-501

[5] Ballantyne GH, Brandner MD, Beart RW Jr, llstrup DM. Volvulus of the colon. Incidence and mortality. Ann surg. 1985;202(1):83-92

[6] Bhatnagar BN, Sharma CL, Gautum A, Kakar A, Reddy DC. Gangrenous sigmoid volvulus: a clinical study of 76 patients . Int J Colorectal Dis.2004;19(2):134-42

[7] Bystrom J, Backman L, Dencker H , Medin-Brith G. Volvulus of the cecum. An analysis of 40 cases and the value of various surgical measures. Acta Chir Scand. 1972;138(6):624-7
[8] Catalano O. Computed tomographic appearance of sigmoid volvulus. Abdom Imaging. 1996;21(4):314-7
[9] Feldman D. The coffee bean sign. Radiology.2000;216(1):178-9
[10] Halliday KE, Bellamy E, Ellis BW. Volvulus of splenic flexure and spleen.Eur Surg.1993;159:383-4
[11] Horgan PG, Gorey TF. Operative assessment of intestinal viability. Surg Clin North Am. 1992;72(1):143-55
[12] Kuzu MA, Aslar AK, Soran A, Polat A, Topcu O, Hengirmen S. Emergent resection for acute sigmoid volvulus: results in 106 consecutive cases. Dis Colon Rectum.2002;45(8):1085-90
[13] Lord SA, Boswell WC, Hungerpillar JC. Sigmoid volvulus in pregnancy. Am Surg.1996;62:380-2
[14] Madiba TE, Thomas SR. The management of cecal volvulus. Dis Colon Rectum.2002;45(2):264-7
[15] Majeski J. Operative therapy for cecal volvulus combining resection with colopexy. Am J Surg.2005;189(2):211-13
[16] Mellor MF, Drake DG. Colonic Volvulus in children : value of barium enema for diagnosis and treatment in the children. AJR. Am J Roentgenol.1994;162(5):1157-9
[17] Mittal R, Samarasam I, Chandran S, Mathew G. Primary splenic flexure volvulus. Singapore Med J.2007;48(3):87-9
[18] Osuka A, Ikegami R, Watanabi Y. Splenic flexure volvulus in a child with chronic idiopathic intestinal pseudo-obstruction syndrome. Pediatr Surg Int.2006;22(10):833-35
[19] Oren D, Atamanalp SS, Aydinli B, Yildirgan MI, Basoglu M, Polat KY, Onbas O. An algorithm for the management of sigmoid colon volvulus and the safety of primary resection. Experience with 827 cases. Dis Colon Rectum.2007;50(4):489-97
[20] Pahlman I, Enblad P, Rudberg C, Krog M. Volvulus of the colon. A review of 93 cases and current aspects of treatment. Acta Chir Scand. 1989;155(1):53-6
[21] Patel A, Kaleya RN, Sammartano RJ. Pathophysiology of mesenteric ischemia. Surg Clin North Am.1992;72(1):31-41
[22] Puthu D, Rajan N, Shenoy GM, Pai US. The ileosigmoid knot. Dis Colon Rectum.1991;34(2):161-6
[23] Raveenthiran V. The ileosigmoid knot: new observations and changing trends. Dis Colon Rectum. 2001;44(8):1196-200
[24] Shepherd JJ. Ninety two cases of ileosigmoid knotting in Uganda. Br J Surg. 1967;54(6):561-6
[25] Tejler G, Jiborn H. Volvulus of the cecum . Report of 26 cases and review of the literature. Dis Colon Rectum. 1988;31:445-90
[26] Zimmerman BJ. Granger DN. Reperfusion injury. Surg Clin North Am. 1992; 72(1):65-83

Part 3

Diabetic Foot, Gangrenous Lung Disease and HIV-Induced Gangrene

Gangrene Associated with Human Immunodeficiency Virus (HIV)

Malladi VSS[1], Abkari S[2] and Srinivasan VR[1]
[1]*Nizam's Institute of Medical Sciences, Hyderabad,*
[2]*Aware Global Hospital, Hyderabad,*
India

1. Introduction

The common aetiologies of gangrene of the extremities are atherosclerosis and diabetes mellitus. An internist may encounter several other diseases which can cause gangrene of extremities. Systemic lupus erythematosus, progressive systemic sclerosis, Henoch-Schonlein purpura, anti-neutrophil cytoplasmic antibody (ANCA) associated vasculitis, Takayasu arteriitis, infective endocarditis, gangrene associated with procoagulant states due to malignancy, anticardiolipin antibody syndrome and disseminated intravascular coagulation are some of the important causes of gangrene of the extremities. Rare causes of gangrene include heparin induced thrombocytopenia (HIT), haemolytic uremic syndrome (HUS) and Human immunodeficiency virus (HIV) infection.

HIV infection involves all the systems of the body, and the cardiovascular system is no exception. HIV vasculopathy was first described as an entity in 1987 (Joshi et al., 1987). HIV associated vasculopathy may present with arterial occlusive disease, aneurysmal disease, aortic dissection or spontaneous arteriovenous fistula (Mulaudzi, 2005; Nair, 1999, 2000, 2001; Pantula, 2009). Vasculitis is one of the less common but important consequences of HIV (Chetty, 2001). Aneursymal disease is thought to be due to vasculitis of vasa vasorum leading to inflammation with resultant transmural fibrosis or necrosis and the formation of true or false aneurysms (Mulauldzi et al., 2005). HIV-related thrombosis, which is segmental, shows a histological picture identical to that seen in aneurysms, with inflammatory changes confined to the vasa vasora with bland organising luminal thrombosis. This strongly suggests that aneurysm and thrombosis are different expressions of the same pathological process.

Peripheral arterial disease (PAD) is more prevalent in the HIV-infected population than in the general population (Periard, 2008). There is a six-fold increased risk for PAD in HIV-infected individuals as well as an earlier onset of the disease compared with HIV-negative patients (Periard et al., 2008). Broad spectrum of rheumatic syndromes are associated with HIV infection ranging from arthralgias to reactive arthritis, myopathy and fibromyalgia to more severe necrotizing vasculitis (Uppal & Achutan, 1997). Almost every pattern and type of vasculitis of small, medium and large vessels has been encountered in the HIV setting (Chetty, 2001). Widespread digital ischemic changes and gangrene of the hands and feet is an uncommon presentation in patients with HIV infection (Roh & Gertner, 1997). There are several reports on HIV associated occlusive vasculopathy from Africa. Reports from India on this subject are limited.

2. Materials and methods

Data of 1311 HIV reactive patients was obtained retrospectively from the medical records of department of medicine from the year 2000 to 2010. All HIV positive patients' records were studied. Records of patients with gangrene were identified and studied.

HIV testing was done by HIV Vironostika (4th Generation ELISA, BioMerieux, France). All HIV reactive samples were then tested by HIV TRIDOT (J Mitra, India), a rapid assay that allows differentiation between HIV 1 and 2. The reactive samples were further confirmed by a Western Blot assay (HIV Blot 2.2, Gene labs Diagnostics, USA). CD4 counts were determined by using the FACS Count (Becton Dickinson, USA). HIV Viral loads were estimated by the AMPLICOR assay (Roche, USA).

3. Our experience

In our experience over the last 10 years in a south Indian tertiary care hospital we have seen only 2 cases of HIV associated gangrene out of the 1311 cases HIV infected patients. We describe our experience of one of our patients of HIV infection with gangrene.

3.1 Case report

A woman aged 32 years presented to the outpatient department of our institute with complaints of pain and blackish discoloration of left foot since 1 month. She did not have diabetes mellitus or hypertension. She was non smoker and non alcoholic. There was no history of coronary artery disease or cerebrovascular diseases.

On examination she was emaciated. Pallor and oral thrush were noted. There was no lymphadenopathy. Vitals were normal. Cardiovascular, abdomen and respiratory systems were normal. Left foot was dry, gangrenous with blackish discoloration (Figure 1). Dorsalis pedis, posterior tibial pulses were not palpable. Sensations decreased on the foot. Hemoglobin was 10 gm/dL, Total leucocyte count was 10,000/cmm with neutrophils 66%, lymphocytes 28%, Eosinophils 4%, and monocytes 2%. Platelets were normal. Peripheral smear examination showed normocytic, normochromic anemia. Erythrocyte sedimentation rate was 20mm at 1st hour. Liver function tests and renal function tests were normal. Lipid profile was normal. Anti nuclear factor (ANF), perinuclear and cytoplasmic anti neutrophil cytoplasmic antibodies (P and C-ANCA) were negative. Australian Antigen and HCV antibodies were negative.

She was evaluated and was found to have HIV-1 infection. CD4 count was 106 cells/μL. Patient's spouse was tested reactive for HIV 1 and was receiving HAART. She had one male child who was 8 years old and had been tested non reactive for HIV infection. She was started on highly active antiretroviral therapy (HAART) and low dose prednisolone. Pain reduced and a line of demarcation developed.

4. Discussion

HIV-associated vascular disease is a specific disease entity which differs from atherosclerotic disease in various aspects. HIV positive patients with vasculopathy are younger with an average age of 40 years in comparison to 55 years in patients with atherosclerotic disease (Botes & Van Marle, 2007). There is also a lower incidence of the typical risk factors for atherosclerosis like smoking, hypertension, hypercholesterolemia and diabetes mellitus in these patients with HIV with peripheral vascular disease. CD4 T-cell

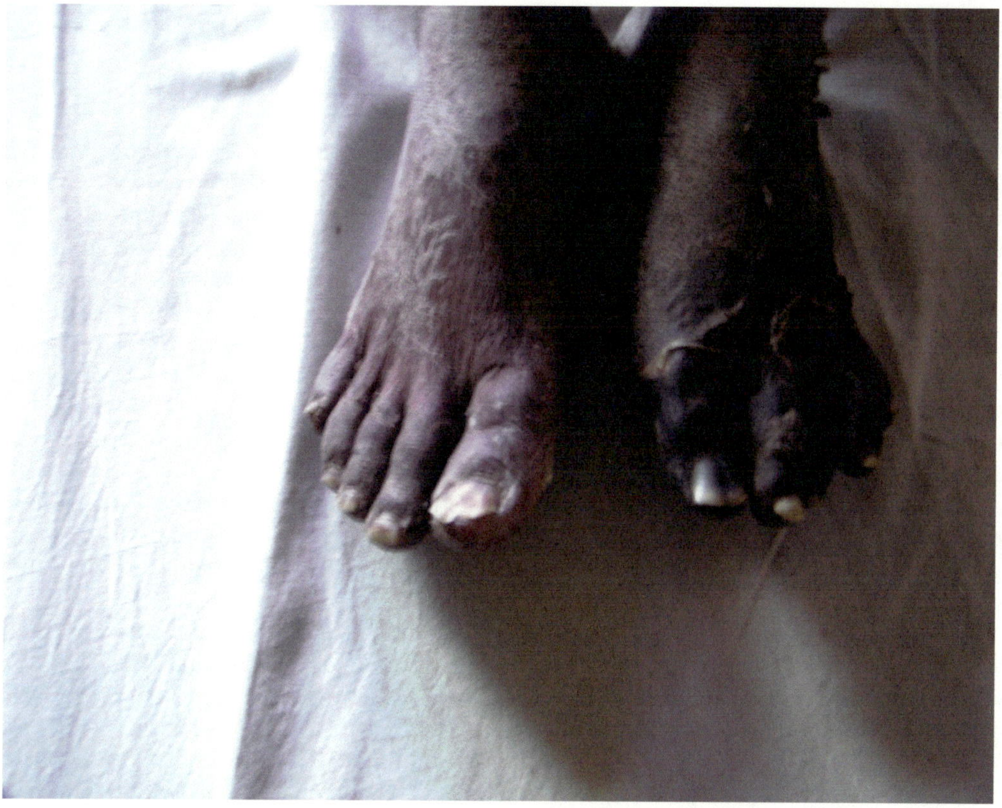

Fig. 1. Gangrene involving left foot in a woman aged 32 years with HIV infection

count < 200 cells/µl was found as significant predictor of PAD in HIV (Periard et al., 2008). Literature suggests that the incidence of symptomatic vasculitis is in the region of 0.4% to 1% of HIV-infected patients (Kaye, 1996; Kakrani et al., 2003). However, we have seen only 2 cases of HIV associated gangrene over last 10 years. The reason for the low incidence in our experience is possibly due to the free antiretroviral treatment (ART) at the government funded ART centres in our state. Another reason for the low incidence of peripheral vascular disease is because we did not screen for any subclinical vascular disease in our patients. As observed in our cases CD4 counts in patients with HIV vasculopathy are below normal in more than 90% of patients and the CD4:CD8 ratio is usually reversed, indicative of advanced immunosuppression (Mulaudzi et al., 2005).

4.1 Etiology of gangrene in HIV

Infections, occlusive disease due to a hypercoagulable state, vasculitis are some of the mechanisms suggested for gangrene of the extremities in HIV. There have been reported findings of anti-phospholipid antibody syndrome, deficiencies of free protein S, protein C and anti-thrombin 3, but these have been sporadic reports. Chronic HIV infection, rather than its pharmacologic treatment, induces alterations of markers of endothelial dysfunction (Torriani et al 2008). However some opine that despite minimizing HIV plasma burden and subsequent associated inflammatory damage, antiretroviral medications may independently contribute to endothelial damage (Gaetano et al., 2003; Chai et al., 2005; Shankar et al., 2005).

HIV-infected patients tend to develop decreases in high density lipoprotein cholesterol (HDL-c) and low density lipoprotein cholesterol (LDL-c) levels, followed by an increase in plasma triglyceride levels, independent of any exposure to antiretroviral therapy (Grunfeld et al., 1992).
Viral infections have been implicated in the pathogenesis of systemic vasculitis, and many viruses, including HIV, are associated with vasculitis and occasionally gangrene. As in any immunocompromised state, opportunistic infections are likely in patients with HIV infection. Vasculitis and gangrene may be a manifestation of these opportunistic infections. Cytomegalovirus (CMV), *Herpes zoster virus* (HZV), toxoplasmosis, pneumocystis, salmonella, and *Mycobacterium tuberculosis* have all been associated with vasculitis in patients with HIV infection[1]. The two major mechanisms by which infection is thought to induce a vasculitis are direct microbial invasion, with resultant damage of the vessel wall, and immune mediated injury both humoral and cellular (Chetty, 2001).
Another mechanism for development of vasculitis in patients after start of antiretroviral therapy (ART) is immune-reconstitution inflammatory syndrome (IRIS). IRIS occurs within a few weeks to months after the start of HAART; patients most often present with clinical deterioration while the number of CD4 lymphocytes is increasing and the HIV viral load decreasing. IRIS could be implicated in the pathogenesis of the vascular complications (Venkataramana et al., 2006).
Various abnormalities predisposing to a hypercoagulable state have been detected in HIV patients, including antiphospholipid antibodies, lupus anticoagulant, increased Von Willebrand factor (vWF), deficiency in protein C and S, antithrombin and heparin co-factor. Viral-induced endothelial injury causes increased levels of Von Willebrand factor, total antigenic protein S, plasminogen activator inhibitor (PAI-1), endothelial-derived thrombomodulin and other procoagulant products of endothelial cell activation (Saif et al., 2001). Some of the rare causes which contribute to gangrene in HIV include thrombotic thrombocytopenic purpura (de Man et al., 1997).

4.2 Clinical features

HIV-associated arterial occlusive disease is recognised as a specific clinical entity. Median age of patients is between 30 - 40 years (Mulaudzi et al., 2005). Male preponderance has been observed in HIV associated vasculopathy (Mulaudzi et al., 2005). The vessels reported to be commonly affected are arteries of muscles and digits. In HIV related occlusive vascular disease two patterns of presentation have been reported (Robbs & Paruk, 2010). In the first type, there is no antecedent claudication and patients present with acute thrombosis. In this type angiographically, proximal vessels appear normal but there is segmental occlusion with poor distal runoff. The second group with occlusive disease appears to have premature atherosclerotic disease. The majority of the patients present with critical ischaemia with rest pain or gangrene.
In most patients the disease is confined to one limb, for reasons that are obscure. However there are case reports describing gangrene involving upper limbs in children with HIV (Despina et al., 2008). Cases of polyarteritis nodosa (PAN) like systemic necrotizing vasculitis in HIV infected individuals, with digital ischaemia are reported (Kakrani et al., 2003). As vasculopathies occur during the later stages of the HIV disease process and are a marker for advanced disease, a thorough search for opportunistic infections should be made in these patients. There are reports of increase in prevalence of Fournier's gangrene in patients with HIV in their surgical ward during post HIV era (Elem& Ranjan, 1995). There

are case reports from India on gangrene involving unusual sites like breast in HIV patients (Venkatramani et al., 2009.)

4.3 Diagnosis

HIV associated gangrene may be associated with a known pathogen or trigger, or may occur in the absence of an obvious identifiable agent. To establish an opportunistic infection associated with the vascular pathology either a serological test, staining of smears on light microscopy, cultures, immunohistochemistry testing , and in situ hybridisation tests or viral markers may be done as are relevant based on the clinical presentation.

Work up for autoimmune diseases and procoagulant states- antinuclear antibodies, antiphospholipd antibodies, protein C, S and anti- thrombin III need to be planned in patients with HIV with gangrene. Patients with peripheral arterial disease can be easily and reliably identified by ankle brachial index (ABI) testing, and they presumably are at increased cardiovascular risk, assuming that ABI mortality correlations from the general population can be extrapolated to HIV-infected persons (Periard et al., 2008).

Doppler study of arterial and venous system is essential in all patients with ischemic changes. There is a pathognomonic sign with hypoechoic spotting within the arterial wall best described as string of pearls sign (Woolgar et al., 2002).

Diagnostic angiography in known HIV-positive patients with vasculopathy requires awareness of the manifestations of the disease (Scholtz, 2004). The uncommon sites and multiplicity of vascular involvement usually imply that additional images, with an increased volume of contrast media, will be required. Owing to the increased risk of thrombosis, care should be taken to adequately heparinize these patients during diagnostic or interventional procedures. In a series on vascular involvement in HIV patients, it was noted that the majority of the patients presented with occlusive disease, followed by aneurysms, usually atypical in location, multiple, clustered and with a predilection for the extracranial carotid arteries followed by the thoracoabdominal aorta and superficial femoral arteries(Sholtz, 2004). Angiographic appearances vary in the two types of HIV related occlusive vascular disease. In the acute thrombosis group, the angiographic picture is one in which the proximal vessels are normal, accompanied by aggressive peripheral thrombotic occlusion and very poor distal runoff.

A careful clinicopathological correlation is particularly important in skin biopsies showing a vasculitic reaction. There are five patterns of vasculitis described in HIV i.e. lymphocytic vasculitis(LyV), leucocytoclastic vasculitis(LCV) of small dermal vessels, neutrophilic vasculitis with vascular thrombosis and intradermal suppuration, vasculitis with palisaded neutrophilic neutrophilic and granulomatous dermatitis and large vessel vasculitis affecting subcutaneous vessels (Grayson, 2008).

The last three patterns usually infer systemic involvement. A neutrophilic (leucocytoclastic) vasculopathic reaction in the HIV positive individual may have many potential causes, including infection with HIV per se. Other viral causes of hypersensitivity vasculitis include CMV, hepatitis B virus, and Epstein–Barr virus. The dermal vessels in skin biopsies from cases of HSV or varicella zoster virus (VZV) infection frequently exhibit LCV. Recurrent varicella may even manifest with vasculitis in the absence of epidermal involvement. Drugs that may precipitate LCV include certain HAART agents, penicillin and the sulphonamides. The presence of acute LCV in association with vascular occlusion may signify either HIV-associated mixed cryoglobulinaemia (with small vessel occlusion by cryoglobulin precipitates) or septic vasculitis (with dermal vascular occlusion by infected microthrombi). The latter may be associated with intradermal abscess formation and/or cutaneous infarction (Carlson, 2005).

4.4 Management

HIV-associated vasculopathy is not cited in the World Health Organization (WHO) clinical staging system. As HIV associated vasculopathy and gangrene are pointers to an advanced stage of the disease it would be logical to offer antiretroviral therapy irrespective of the CD4 level. Recent publications have shown that HIV itself as a risk factor for peripheral artery disease and strongly recommended NRTI and NNRTI containing regimens (Ye, 2010). As a class, the protease inhibitors appear to have the greatest negative impact on total cholesterol and triglyceride levels; however, even within this class, certain agents e.g., atazanivir and darunavir do not have an adverse effect on lipids.

The treatment in patients with acute thrombosis type of occlusive disease depends on the clinical presentation. In those patients wherein the limb cannot be salvaged primary amputation is done. Where the limb is salvageable treatment options include endovascular procedures like thrombectomy and thrombolysis or bypass procedures. However, the limb salvage rate has been in the region of 27% (Mulaudzi et al., 2005). This is thought to be due to the fact that it is mainly a vasculitic process with superimposed thrombosis, and removing the thrombus does not, in effect, solve the problem, which has a very high re-thrombosis rate[3].

Patients with HIV infection with widespread ischemic necrosis and gangrene may require treatment with corticosteroids (in the event of possible vasculitis), thrombolytic agents (for the thrombotic component), or both, unless there are contraindications to either (Roh & Gertner, 1997).

In those with chronic occlusive type of disease, in almost half of the patients, there may not be a possibility of reconstruction due to poor runoff or the limb may be beyond salvage. In others standard bypass procedures can be performed and only recently have endovascular procedures been attempted. In this group, the results are marginally better than in the patients with acute thrombosis type of occlusive disease. (Robbs & Paruk, 2010).

Patients should be optimized as per standard practice prior to surgical or endovascular intervention. Vascular surgical principles should be adhered to when managing patients with HIV-associated occlusive vasculopathy and management should be individualized. Various authors have identified a CD4 T-cell count of less than 200 cells/µl is an important risk factor for postoperative complications (Lin et al., 2004; Albaran, et al., 1998). A significant complication in all patients in whom surgery is attempted has been the high rate of superficial wound sepsis and graft sepsis. Some centers with vast experience with surgical procedures for occlusive vascular disease in HIV have reported a perioperative mortality of 6.95% (Van Marle et al., 2009). Primary amputation is usually done for very advanced arterial disease.

5. Conclusions

One of the unforeseen consequences of untreated long standing infection with HIV is the appearance of various rheumatic syndromes. Clinicians encountering a patient with gangrene should consider HIV as an important cause and screen for presence of HIV antibodies. Early detection of the HIV infection and appropriate and timely start of HAART can possibly prevent vascular complications. In every patient, workup for both traditional and specific risk factors including opportunistic infections and prothrombotic states should be done. Appropriate treatment for the ischemic limb as well as treatment of opportunistic infections and HAART when indicated may significantly improve the outcomes. Screening for subclinical vascular disease in asymptomatic patients with simple measures like ankle brachial index and appropriate timely treatment will go a long way in preventing the development of gangrene.

6. Acknowledgements

I sincerely thank my husband Dr. P. Narasingarao, Cardiac Surgeon at Kamineni Hospital, King Koti for the support and guidance during the preparation of the manuscript.

7. References

Albaran, RG.; Webber, J., & Steffes, CP. (1998). CD4 cell counts as a prognostic factor of major abdominal surgery in patients infected with the human immunodeficiency virus. *Arch Surg,* Vol. 133, pp. 626-631.

Botes, K. & Van Marle, J. (2007). Surgical Intervention for HIV Related Vascular Disease. *Eur J Vasc Endovasc Surg,* Vol. 34, pp. 390-396.

Carlson, JA.; Ng, BT. & Chen, K-R. (2005). Cutaneous vasculitis update: diagnostic criteria, classification, epidemiology, etiology, pathogenesis, evaluation and prognosis. *Am J Dermatopathol,* Vol. 27, pp. 504–528.

Chai, H.; Yang, H.; Yan, S, *et al.* (2005). Effects of 5 HIV protease inhibitors on vasomotor function and superoxide anion production in porcine coronary arteries. *J Acquir Immune Defic Syndr,* Vol. 40, p. 12.

Chetty, R. (2001). Vasculitides associated with HIV infection. *J Clin Pathol,* Vol. 54, pp. 275-278.

Daniel, Periard.; Matthias, Cavassini; Patrick Taffe, *et al.* (2008). High Prevalence of Peripheral Arterial Disease in HIV-Infected Persons. *Clinical Infectious Diseases,* Vol. 46, pp. 761–767.

de Gaetano, Donati, K.; Rabagliati, R.; Tumbarello, M., *et al.* (2003). Increased soluble markers of endothelial dysfunction in HIV-positive patients under highly active antiretroviral therapy. *AIDS,* Vol. 17, p. 765.

de Man, AM.; Smulders, YM.; Roozendaal, KJ., *et al.* (1997). HIV-related thrombotic thrombocytopenic purpura: report of 2 cases and a review of the literature. *Neth J Med,* Vol. 51, pp. 103-109.

Despina, Demopoulos; Hendson, W.; Technau, K., *et al.* (2009). Vasculopathy in HIV-infected children - a case series. *S Afr J CH,* Vol. 3, pp. 27-30.

Elem, B.; & Ranjan, P. (1995). Impact of Immunodeficiency virus (HIV) on Fournier's gangrene: observations in Zambia. *Ann R Coll Surg Engl,* Vol. 77, pp. 283-286.

Grayson, W. (2008). The HIV-positive skin biopsy. *J Clin Pathol, Vol.* 61, pp. 802-817.

Grunfeld, C.; Pang, M.; Doerrler, W. & Shigenaga, JK. (1992) Lipids, lipoproteins, triglyceride clearance and cytokines in human immunodeficiency virus infection and the acquired immunodeficiency syndrome. *J Clin Endocrinol Metab,* Vol. 74, p. 1045.

Joshi, VV.; Pawel, B.; Connor, E., *et al.* (1987). Arteriopathy in children with acquired immunodeficiency syndrome. *Pediatr Pathol,* Vol. 7, pp. 261-275.

Kakrani, AL.; Anita Basavraj, R; Madraki. (2003). Vasculitis with digital gangrene in a patient with HIV Infection. *J Assoc Physicians India,* Vol. 51, pp.299-301.

Kaye, B. (1996). Rheumatologic manifestations of HIV infections. *Clin Rev Allergy Immunol,* Vol. 14, pp. 385-416.

Leonie Scholtz. (2004). Vascular Manifestations of HIV/AIDS. *Cardiovasc Intervent Radiol,* Vol. 27, pp. 422–426.

Lin, PH.; Bush, RL.; Yao, Q, *et al.* (2004). Abdominal aortic surgery in patients with human immunodeficiency virus infection. *Am J Surg,* Vol. 188, pp. 690-697.

Mulaudzi, TV.; Robbs, JV.; Pillay, W, *et al.* (2005). Thrombectomy in HIV related peripheral arterial thrombosis: a preliminary report. *Eur J Vasc Endovasc Surg,* Vol. 30, No.1, pp. 102-106.

Nair, R.; Abdool-Carrim, ATO.; Chetty R., *et al.* (1999). Arterial aneurysm in patients infected with human immunodeficiency virus: a distinct clinicopathology entity? *J Vasc Surg,* Vol. 29, pp. 600-607.

Nair, R.; Chetty, R. ; Woolgar, J., *et al.* (2001). Spontaneous arteriovenous fistula resulting from HIV arteritis. *J Vasc Surg,* Vol. 3, No.1, pp. 186-187.

Nair, R.; Robbs, JV.; Chetty, R., *et al.* (2000). Occlusive arterial disease in HIV-infected patients: a preliminary report. *Eur J Vasc Endovasc Surg,* Vol. 20, pp. 353-357.

Narasinga Rao Pantula, & Malladi Venkata Surya Subbalaxmi. (2009). Repair of aortic dissection in a patient with advanced AIDS. *Ind J Thorac Cardiovasc Surg,* Vol. 25, pp. 65-67.

Periard, D.; Cavassini, M.; Taffé, P., *et al.* (2008). High prevalence of peripheral arterial disease in HIV-infected persons. *HIV/AIDS CID,* Vol. 46, pp. 761-767.

Robbs, JV.;Paruk,N.; (2010) Management of HIV Vasculopathy -A South African Experience. *Eur J Vasc Endovasc Surg* Vol. 39 pp. S25eS31.

Roh, SS., & Gertner, E. (1997). Digital necrosis in acquired immune deficiency syndrome vasculopathy treated with recombinant tissue plasminogen activator. *J Rheumatol,* Vol. 24, pp. 2258-2261.

Saif, MW.; Bona, R.; & Greenberg, B. (2001). AIDS and thrombosis: Retrospective study of 131 HIV-infected patients. *AIDS Patient Care and STDs,* Vol. 15, pp. 311-320.

Shankar, SS.; Dube, MP.; Gorski, JC., *et al.* (2005). Indinavir impairs endothelial function in healthy HIV-negative men. *Am Heart J,* Vol. 150, p. 933.

Torriani, FJ.; Komarow, L.; Parker, RA., *et al.* (2008). Endothelial function in human immunodeficiency virus-infected antiretroviral-naive subjects before and after starting potent antiretroviral therapy: The ACTG (AIDS Clinical Trials Group) Study 5152s. *J Am Coll Cardiol,* Vol. 52, p. 569.

Uppal, SS., & Achutan, K. (1997). Impact of HIV infection on rheumatic diseases. *J Assoc Physicians India,* Vol. 45, pp. 387-391.

Van Marle, J.; Mistry, PP., & Botes, K. (2009). Vascular disease in HIV/AIDS.*SAJS,* Vol. 47, pp. 37-42.

Venkataramana, A.; Pardo, CA., McArthur, JC, *et al.* (2006). Immune reconstitution inflammatory syndrome in CNS of HIV- infected patients. *Neurology,* Vol. 67, pp. 383-388.

Venkatramani, V.; Pillai, S.; Marathe, S; *et al.* (2009). Breast gangrene in an HIV-positive patient *AnnR Coll Surg Engl* Vol. 91, pp.1-2.

Woolgar, JD.; Ray, R.; Maharaj, K., *et al.* (2002). Colour Doppler and grey scale ultrasound features of HIV-related vascular aneurysm. *Br J Radiol,* Vol. 75, pp. 884-888.

Yikong, Ye; Yong Zeng; Xiaomeng Li, *et al.* (2010). HIV infection: An independent risk factor of peripheral artery disease. *J Acquir Immune Defic Syndr,* Vol. 53, pp. 276-278.

10

Gangrenous Lung Disease

Chih-Hao Chen
Department of Thoracic Surgery, Mackay Memorial Hospital, Taipei City, Taiwan

1. Introduction

Normal lung function requires both adequate lung ventilation and adequate perfusion. Adequate lung perfusion means normal blood flow can reach to the lung tissues providing nutrients and oxygen to the lung tissues and the waste can be removed. Perfusion of the lung may be disturbed in numerous settings, including infection, aspiration of foreign body, neoplasm[1], trauma and may be secondary to surgical complications, adverse effects of radiation therapy and chemotherapeutic agents. A variety of causes may lead to gangrenous lung disease.(Table 1) For example, uncontrolled diabetes is a risk factor of severe lung infection, especially caused by *Klebsiella* pneumonia.[4] Inadequate blood flow usually resulted in necrosis, bacterial overgrowth and abscess formation. Gangrenous change indicates tissues necrosis followed by decomposition of tissues into a slough. Compromise of blood flow can be the primary cause and can be the result of other antecedent events. Treatment and outcome were essentially related to its causes and depends on the timing of either medical or surgical intervention. Without prompt intervention, high risks of mortality and morbidity will be encountered.

Primary		
	pneumonia	severe and uncontrolled infection in lung tissues
	pulmonary embolism	hypercoagulable state, deep vein thrombosis
	neoplasm	lung cancer with necrosis and infection, bronchial obliteration by hilar tumor or hilar lymphadenopathy
Secondary		
	trauma	lung contusional hemorrhage
	surgery	Improper ligation of pulmonary artery and vein, lobar torsion
	sepsis	septic emoli, systemic infection
	drug-induced	lung toxicity of chemotherapeutic agents
	radiation effect	radiation pneumonitis
	foreign body aspiration	aspiration pneumonia

Table 1. Etiology of pulmonary gangrene

2. Clinical features

Inflammatory changes can be locally confined in the lung tissues with lobar pneumonia, necrotizing pneumonitis, cystic changes and abscess occurring in any location where the tissues being destroyed. Symptoms of local inflammatory diseases include chest pain, pleurisy, cough, dyspnea, purulent expectorants and reduced tolerance of physical activity. Systemic inflammatory response syndrome (SIRS) causes unstable hemodynamics (dropped blood pressure, tachycardia, tachypnea / dyspnea, and high fever/chills), severe chest pain, malaise, poor appetite and purulent expectorants. In advanced age patients, deterioration of consciousness may be the first presentation. However, these symptoms may be subtle or non-specific and resembled to those symptoms seen in other common diseases. Characteristic features included abundant and putrid sputum in the airway and hemoptysis caused by tissues decomposition. [2] Proper history taking is essential when the patient presented unexpected presentations following surgery (for example improper pulmonary artery ligation after a lung resection). The diagnosis of lung gangrene based on clinical manifestations alone is quite difficult. Established risk factors of community-acquired pneumonia (CAP) are alcoholism, asthma, immunosuppression, advanced age (> 70 years old), dementia, seizure, congestive heart failure, cerebralvascular disease, chronic obstructive pulmonary disease, smoking, end-stage renal disease and others.[3]

3. Diagnostic laboratory blood test

A complete cell count and biochemistry is mandatory. Elevated white blood cells with shift-to-left usually indicates for systemic inflammation or infection. C-reactive protein, erythrocyte sedimentation rate and procalcitonin are also useful infection indicators. When systemic infection is severe and non-pulmonary origins can be reasonably excluded, gangrenous changes, a form of the most severe lung infection and tissues decomposition, should be kept in mind as one of the differential diagnosis.[3, 5] Blood culture is obtained if bacteremia is likely and serology test will be useful in some instances of infection.

4. Sputum analysis

Obtaining adequate sputum for possible pathogens is essential to guide the use of antibiotics. Prior to identifying the definite culprit pathogen, empiric antibiotics of broad-spectrum should be started as soon as possible. Four common pathogens encountered in community-acquired pneumonia are Streptococcus pneumonia, *Haemophilus* influenzae, *Staphylococcus* aureus and *Mycoplasma* pneumoniae. Among the common pathogens, Streptococcus pneumonia occupied more than 50% of all cases. Gram stain, Acid-fast stain and rapid antigen test can assist differential diagnosis. A positive gram stain for diplococci has near 100% sensitivity for pneumococcal infection but the specificity is poor (less than 5%). [5] Recently, polymerase chain reaction (PCR) becomes more and more popular in detection of some pathogens, from throat swab or sputum, yielding rapid result to guide our treatment strategy. A multiplex PCR allows us to detect tuberculosis, *Legionella* spp, *Mycoplasma* pneumoniae and C. Pneumonia. However, due to higher costs, such test is not routinely applicable.

5. Bronchoscopy

Bronchoscopy is a useful tool to help evaluate the condition of trachea and bronchus. Lobar torsion, most commonly encountered in right middle lobe following resection of right upper lobe, and subsequent lobar gangrene can be diagnosed under bronchoscopic findings of total obliteration of bronchial orifice.[6] Ischemic bronchial wall can also be demonstrated under bronchoscope. With brushing, lavage with saline (BAL) and punch biopsy of suspected endobronchial lesion may also assist proper diagnosis prior to definitive treatment.

6. Images

6.1 Chest radiograph

Chest radiograph can demonstrate disease progression from a smaller pneumonia patch, lobar pneumonia, lung abscess, parapneumonic effusion and then to diffuse necrotic and gangrenous changes of the lung. Consolidation of lung, cavitation and interstitial infiltrates are possible changes. (Figure 1)When clinical suspicion of lung infection is high but chest radiograph is normal, interval follow-up of chest radiograph is mandatory. Many other disease may have similar image findings. As a result, diagnostic value of these findings is quite low.(Figure 1)

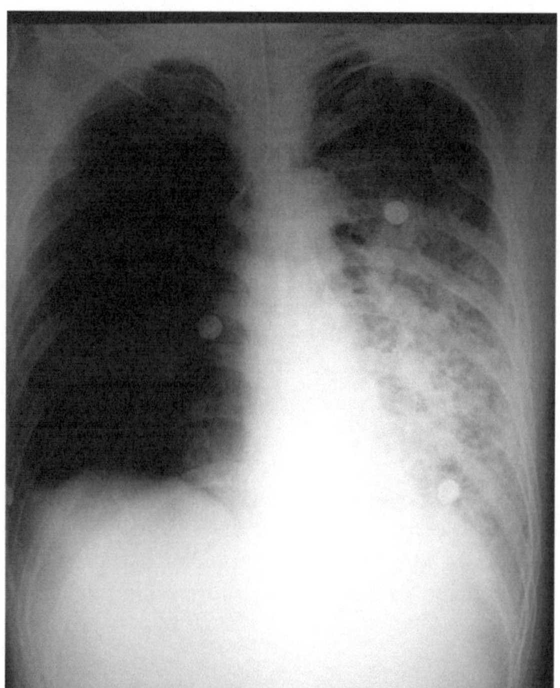

Fig. 1. Chest radiograph showed unilateral involvement of the lung with increased infiltrates and patchy consolidation with apical lung spared.

6.2 Angniography

When normal blood flow to the infected lung had been disturbed, angiography is an adequate methods to evaluate the vascular structure and help differentiate from other diseases. [7] However, pulmonary angiography is an invasive procedure carrying higher risks of vascular injury. In most circumstances, the role of diagnosis has been replaced by CTA (computed-tomography angiography), which is a relatively less invasive approach. [8]

6.3 Computed tomography

Computed tomography (CT) can clearly define gangrenous lung disease into localized form and diffuse form. With and without contrast enhancement can help identify the involved regions, preoperative evaluation for the extent of lung resection, and whether pulmonary vessels are occluded or not. Gangrenous changes of lung on CT scan have features of multiple low-density areas, consolidations, air-trapping, loculated effusion and possibly hydropneumothorax due to broncho-pleural fistula. Figure 2 is an example of the patterns of both consolidation, necrosis and parapneumonic effusion.

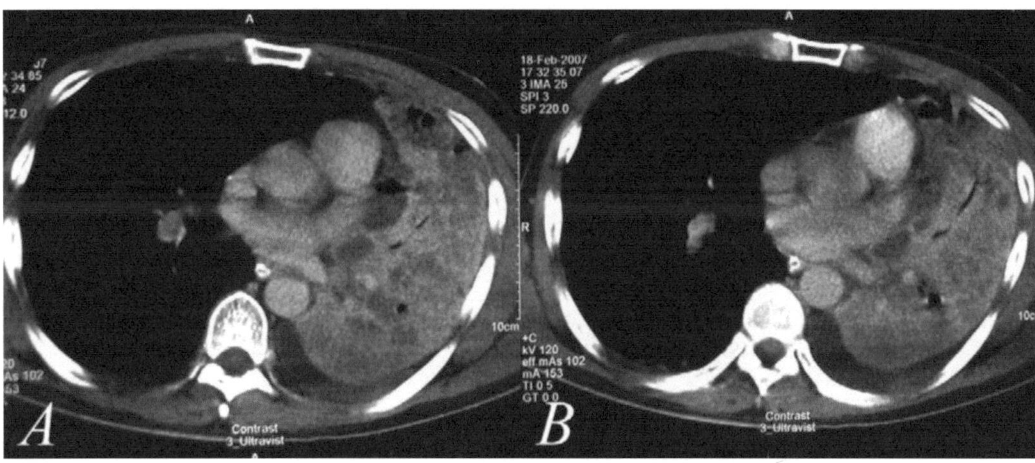

Fig. 2. Computed tomography scan of the lung showed multiple low-density regions with marked consolidation as well as some parapneumonic effusions. The contralateral lung is spared. The involved hemithorax is smaller in volume while the spared hemithorax expands normally.

6.4 Lung function test

Lung function test is not for definite diagnosis but for evaluation the possibility of lung resection and determine the extent of resection. However, the infected lung usually has impaired lung function. Nuclear scan maybe more useful to determine the percentage of lung function of each lobe. Such test can differentiate restrictive lung disease from obstructive lung disease.

6.5 Nuclear imaging

Nuclear scan helps little in establishment of definite diagnosis. However, both perfusion and ventilation scan help a lot in evaluation of the extent of lung resection and estimated post-operative lung function. Lung function test alone can determine the patient's overall lung function but can not predict the function, perfusion and ventilation, of individual lobe and gives us more reliable reading than lung function test alone. However, due to the limitation of resolution of nuclear scan, interpretation of the results should be careful and may discuss with the specialists.

7. Treatment

7.1 Medical treatment

Medical treatment is still the mainstay of treatment of gangrenous lung disease. The goals of medical treatment is to control both local and systemic infection, preventing occurrence of SIRS and septic shock. Administration of broad-spectrum of antibiotics, proper fluid replacement therapy, steroid therapy, secure airway are useful strategies. Emperic antibiotics should be modified according to culture results. When patient's response is poor despite of aggressive medical treatment, surgical evaluation ought to be considered. The most appropriate timing of surgery is to be defined. According to the experience of our institute, after aggressive medical treatment for 48 hrs, surgical evaluation is to be expected to prevent bilateral involvement of necrotizing pneumonia and unavoidable lethal outcome. If patient's condition become stablized and the infected lung was only confined locally. Resection of the local infection can be either delayed or unnecessary depending on infection control.

7.2 Surgical treatment

Adequate timing of surgical intervention isn't easy to determine because gangrenous changes of lung often accompany with pleural infection including empyema thoracis and chest wall infection. Resection of lung, division of pulmonary vessels and bronchus in an infected pleural space is risky for postoperative bleeding, prolonged air leaks due to bronchial rupture and persistent pleural infection. A two-stage approach had been proposed a reasonable strategy.[9] With concomitant pleural space infection, tube thoracostomy to allow drainage of purulent pleural effusion or thoracoscopic deloculation and decortication to help cleaning of pleural space and prepare for subsequent lung resection. However, infection may be overwhelming in some situations and surgical intervention is emergent. The most appropriate timing should be judged individually because such information in the literature is very limited. If tube thoracostomy failed to alleviate systemic infection, prompt surgical intervention should be started. If bronchial or vascular structure is fragile and necrotic, pleural or muscle flap may be considered during operation. Extent of resection is according to the involved lung tissues with normal lung spared. [4] Gross appearance of gangrenous lung may be from densely fibrotic (Figure 3) to very fragile with foul smell. (Figure 4)

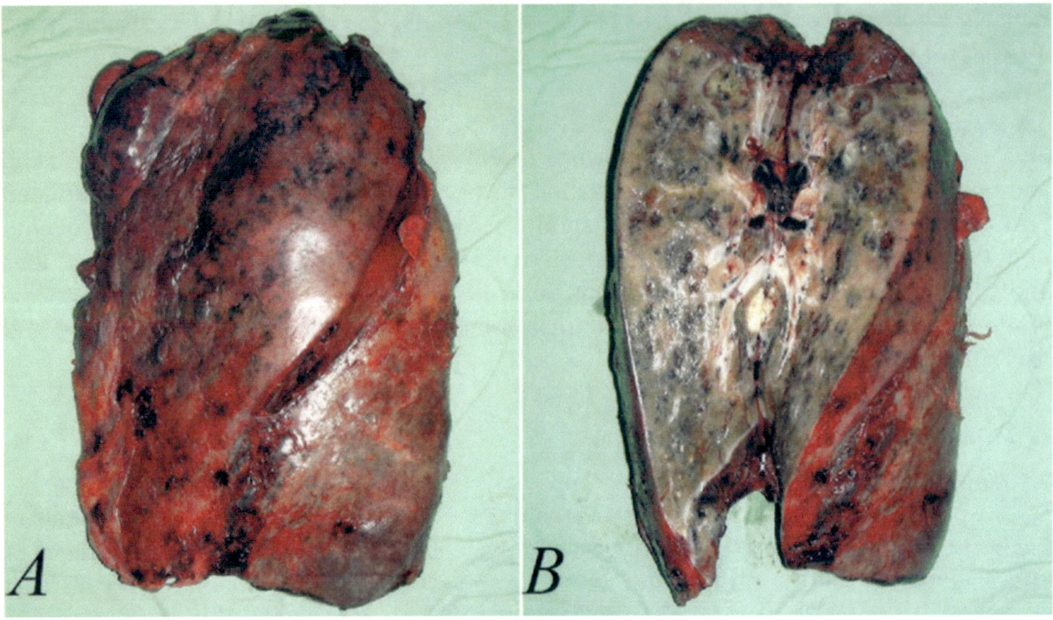

Fig. 3. This is a specimen after left side pneumonectomy. Repeated infection with regeneration will result in consolidation(hepatization) and may cause pulmonary artery occlusion. Such interruption of blood flow further aggravates infection because the antibiotics may not reach to necrotic tissues.

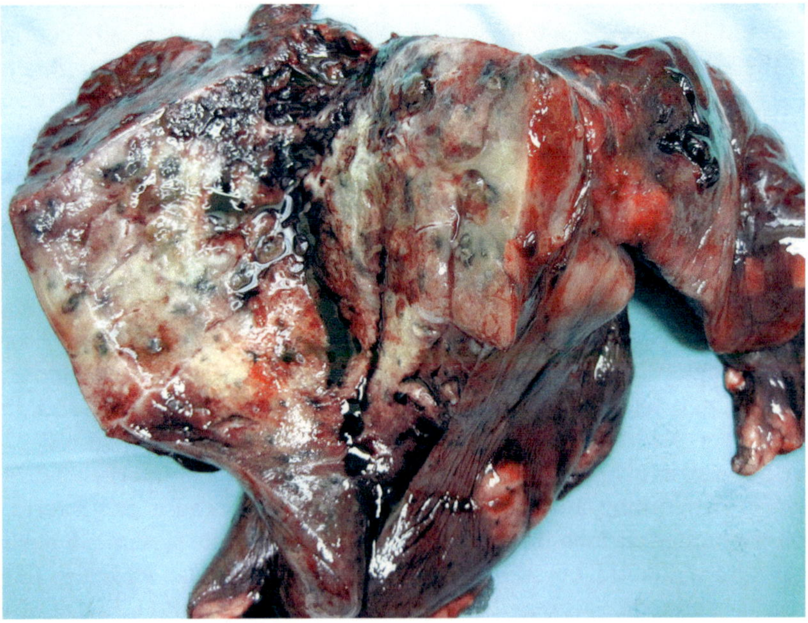

Fig. 4. This is a specimen of right middle and right lower lobe after bilobectomy. On cut, there was foul smell and the lung was very fragile in some regions admixed with some fibrotic regions.

8. ECMO

Extracorporeal membrane oxygenation is a strategy when lung fails to provide adequate level of oxygenation.[10] Whether a patient's condition is operable or can be treated medically, ECMO can maintain adequate oxygenation (V-V mode) and circulation (A-V mode) when lung condition is potentially reversible. Currently, more and more evidences support the role of ECMO in non-cardiac circulatory failure. The exact timing and place of such treatment in lung infection management remains to be determined

8.1 Outcome

Outcome depends mostly on the timing of detection of the gangrenous changes and prompt intervention, either medical or surgical. Currently, there is still no reliable statistical results about the mortality rate and complication rate. In some instances, auto-pneumonectomy may occur after severe infection in hemi-lung without resection. This condition is termed as " dry gangrene" and the involved lung becomes functionless and does not cause further systemic infection. This is only rarely occurred. In most conditions, prompt surgical intervention is mandatory if medical treatment failed to alleviate sepsis within days. When involvement of pulmonary gangrene extends more than one lobe, extent of lung resection need to be carefully evaluated. After complete resection of the necrotic tissues, infection control will be easier. Chest tube can be removed days after operation. Long-term follow-up is mandatory because most patients with pulmonary infections, to the extent of necrosis and gangrene, have obvious predisposing factors and these factors must be monitored carefully in outpatient department. Pulmonary rehabilitation is strongly recommended 3 months after lung resection.

9. Conclusion

In most circumstances, lung infection is a medical disease and rarely requires lung resection. However, surgical intervention should be carefully evaluated when a patient's condition rapidly deteriorates despite aggressive medical treatment.

10. References

[1] Bellido Casado, J., J.L. Carretero Sastre, I. Recio Rueda, A. Smucler Simonovich, and M.A. Torres Nieto, [Trousseau's syndrome in lung adenocarcinoma. The rare appearance of venous gangrene]. Arch Bronconeumol, 1997. 33: 312-4.

[2] Hammond, J.M., C. Lyddell, P.D. Potgieter, and J. Odell, Severe pneumococcal pneumonia complicated by massive pulmonary gangrene. Chest, 1993. 104: 1610-2.

[3] Basi, S.K., T.J. Marrie, J.Q. Huang, and S.R. Majumdar, Patients admitted to hospital with suspected pneumonia and normal chest radiographs: epidemiology, microbiology, and outcomes. Am J Med, 2004. 117: 305-11.

[4] Chen, C.H., W.C. Huang, T.Y. Chen, T.T. Hung, and H.C. Liu, Massive necrotizing pneumonia with pulmonary gangrene. Ann Thorac Surg, 2009. 87: 310-1.

[5] Fine, M.J., T.E. Auble, D.M. Yealy, et al., A prediction rule to identify low-risk patients with community-acquired pneumonia. N Engl J Med, 1997. 336: 243-50.

[6] Chen, C.H., T.T. Hung, T.Y. Chen, and H.C. Liu, Torsion of right middle lobe after a right upper lobectomy. J Cardiothorac Surg, 2009. 4: 16.

[7] Engelke, C., C. Schaefer-Prokop, E. Schirg, et al., High-resolution CT and CT angiography of peripheral pulmonary vascular disorders. Radiographics, 2002. 22: 739-64.
[8] Anderson, J.T., T. Jenq, M. Bain, et al., Diagnosis of posttraumatic pulmonary embolism: is chest computed tomographic angiography acceptable? J Trauma, 2003. 54: 472-7.
[9] Refaely, Y. and D. Weissberg, Gangrene of the lung: treatment in two stages. Ann Thorac Surg, 1997. 64: 970-3; discussion 973-4.
[10] Brenner, M., J.V. O'Connor, and T.M. Scalea, Use of ECMO for resection of post-traumatic ruptured lung abscess with empyema. Ann Thorac Surg, 2010. 90: 2039-41.

11

Diabetic Foot and Gangrene

Jude Rodrigues and Nivedita Mitta
Department of Surgery, Goa Medical College, India

1. Introduction

"Early intervention in order to prevent potential disaster in the management of Diabetic foot is not only a great responsibility, but also a great opportunity"

Despite advances in our understanding and treatment of diabetes mellitus, diabetic foot disease still remains a terrifying problem. Diabetes is recognized as the most common cause of non-traumatic lower limb amputation in the western world, with individuals over 20 times more likely to undergo an amputation compared to the rest of the population. There is growing evidence that the vascular contribution to diabetic foot disease is greater than was previously realised. This is important because, unlike peripheral neuropathy, Peripheral Arterial Occlusive Disease (PAOD) due to atherosclerosis, is generally far more amenable to therapeutic intervention. PAOD, has been demonstrated to be a greater risk factor than neuropathy in both foot ulceration and lower limb amputation in patients with diabetes. Diabetes is associated with macrovascular and microvascular disease. The term peripheral vascular disease may be more appropriate when referring to lower limb tissue perfusion in diabetes, as this encompasses the influence of both microvascular dysfunction and PAOD.

Richards-George P. in his paper about vasculopathy on Jamaican diabetic clinic attendees showed that Doppler measurements of ankle/brachial pressure index (A/BI) revealed that 23% of the diabetics had peripheral occlusive arterial disease (POAD) which was mostly asymptomatic. This underscores the need for regular Doppler A/BI testing in order to improve the recognition, and treatment of POAD. Ageing is associated with both neuropathic ulcers and peripheral vascular diseases among individual with diabetes.

2. Diabetic foot

The foot of a diabetic patient has the potential risk of pathologic consequences, including ulceration, infection and/or destruction of deep tissues associated with neurologic abnormalities, varying degrees of peripheral vascular disease and/or metabolic complications of diabetes in the lower limb.

2.1 Epidemiology and problem statement of diabetic foot

The foot ulcer incidence rates range between 2% and 10% among patients with diabetes mellitus. The age adjusted annual incidence for non traumatic lower limb amputations in diabetic persons ranges form 2.1 to 13.7 per 1000 persons.[1]

It is estimated that 15% of diabetic patients will experience a foot ulcer at some time over the course of their disease. People with foot problems and diabetes mellitus have 15 times the increased risk of undergoing a lower extremity amputation compared to those without diabetes[2]. Amputation is the end result of a cascade of diabetic foot leg lesions. Twenty percent of all diabetic persons enter the hospital because of foot problems. One study in UK showed that 50% of the hospital bed occupancy of diabetic patients is caused by foot problems.
Apart from the morbidity and mortality associated with diabetic foot ulcers and amputations, the economic and emotional consequences for the patient and the family can be enormous[3].

2.2 Classification of the diabetic foot[4]

For practical purposes, the diabetic foot can be divided into two entities, the neuropathic foot and the ischaemic foot. However, ischaemia is nearly always associated with neuropathy, and the ischaemic foot is best called the neuroischaemic foot. The purely ischaemic foot, with no concomitant neuropathy, is rarely seen in diabetic patients.

2.2.1 The neuropathic foot

- It is a warm, well perfused foot with bounding pulses due to arteriovenous shunting and distended dorsal veins.
- Sweating is diminished, the skin may be dry and prone to fissuring
- Toes may be clawed and the foot arch raised.
- Ulceration commonly develops on the sole of the foot
- Despite the good circulation, necrosis can develop secondary to severe infection.
- It is also prone to bone and joint problems (the charcot foot).

2.2.2 The neuroischaemic foot

- It is a cool, pulseless foot with reduced perfusion and invariably has neuropathy.
- The colour of the severely ischaemic foot can be a deceptively healthy pink or red, caused by dilatation of capillaries in an attempt to improve perfusion. If severely infected, the ischaemic foot may feel deceptively warm.
- It may also be complicated by swelling, often secondary to cardiac or renal failure.
- The most frequent presentation is that of ulceration. Ischaemic ulcers are commonly seen on the margin of the foot, which includes the tips of the toes and the areas around the back of the heel, and are usually caused by trauma or by wearing unsuitable shoes
- Intermittent claudication and rest pain may be absent because of neuropathy and the distal distribution of the arterial disease of the leg.
- Even if neuropathy is present and plantar pressures are high, plantar ulceration is rare,
- It develops necrosis in the presence of infection or if tissue perfusion is critically diminished.

2.3 The natural history of the diabetic foot :

The natural history of the diabetic foot can be divided into six stages
Stage 1 : Normal - Not at risk. The patient does not have the risk factors of neuropathy, ischemia, deformity, callus and swelling rendering him/her vulnerable to foot ulcers.
Stage 2 : High risk foot – the patient has developed one or more of the risk factors for ulceration of the foot.

Stage 3 : Ulcerated foot – the foot has a skin breakdown. This is usually an ulcer, but because some minor injuries such as blisters, splits or grazes have a propensity to become ulcers, they are included in stage 3.
Stage 4 : Infected foot – the ulcer has developed infection with the presence of cellulitis.
Stage 5 : Necrotic foot – necrosis has supervened.
Stage 6 : Unsalvageable – The foot cannot be saved and will need a major amputation.

2.4 Pathogenesis of diabetic foot lesions[5]

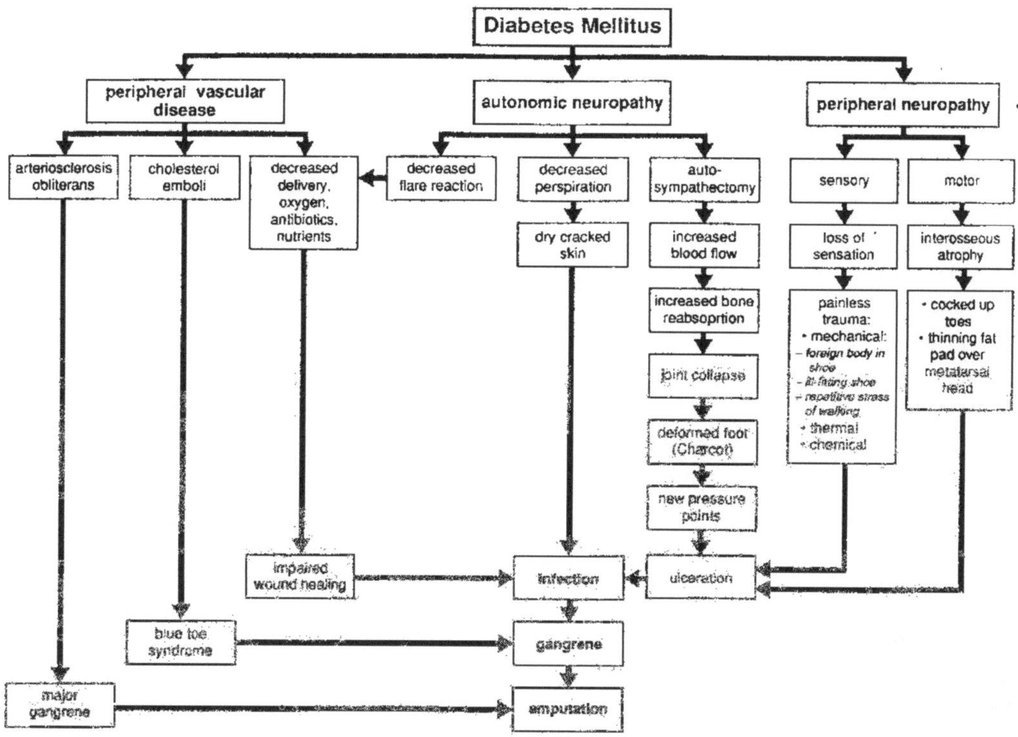

3. Pathophysiology

Recent advances in molecular biology have added substantial insight into the pathophysiology of the disease and opened new avenues for treatment[1].
The predisposing factors to pathologic changes in the foot of a diabetic are

1. Metabolic factors – hyperglycemia
2. Vascular changes
3. Neuropathy
4. Infection

3.1 Metabolic factors

Hyperglycemia is the common feature in the two etiologic types of diabetes[2]. Hyperglycemia influences the development of complication of diabetes through the following metabolic pathways.

a. Polyol pathway:

Glucose ⟶ Sorbitol ⟶ accumulation in nerves, retina, kidneys.

Hyperglycemia results in increased levels of sorbitol in the cell, which acts like an osmolyte a competitive inhibitor of myoinositol uptake. This preferential shunting of glucose through the sorbitol pathway results in decreased mitochondrial pyruvate utilization and decreased energy production. This process is termed "Hyperglycemia induced pseudohypoxia."

b. Glycation of proteins:

Glucose + protein amino group

↓

Early glycosylation products (poorly irreversible)

↓

Advanced glycosylation products (completely irreversible)

↙ ↓ ↘

Endothelium	Macrophages	Extra cellular matrix protein
↑Procoagulant Activity ↑Permeability ↑Activation of NF-KB	↑Chemotaxis ↑Growth Factor synthesis ↑Monokinins secretion	↑Cross linking of collagen ↑Trapping of serum proteins (LDL) ↑Susceptibility to enzymatic degradation

3.2 Vascular changes

Involvement of the blood vessels by atherosclerosis leading to ischaemia is a significant factor in diabetic foot. Lower extremity peripheral vascular disease (PVD) is the most common factor associated with limb ulceration gangrene, impaired wound healing and ultimately amputation[2].

It mainly occurs in

a. blood flow changes
b. occlusive changes
c. micro angiopathy
d. hematological changes

Blood flow changes: There is marked change in the flow of blood in peripheral vessels. The microcirculation is regulated by neural factors, local reflexes and vasoactive mediators. The initial haemodynamic changes will be increased flow and pressure of capillary blood[9]. As the disease progresses, autoregulation is lost and haemodynamic stress results. It could also be due to increased calcification of vessels or AV shunting or hyperosmolarity of blood. It is well documented by high ankle brachial ratio and also Doppler studies.

Occlusive changes: More than 50% of diabetics having the disease for more than 10 - 15 years are documented to have atherosclerotic changes[6]. It mainly affects arteries below profunda femoris and is characterized by multiple segment involvement. The tibial & peroneal arteries between the knee and the ankle are primarily affected. Dorsalis pedis artery and foot vessels are usually spared. Patients with diabetes have diminished ability to establish collateral circulation especially in arteries around knee[2]. Atherosclerotic vascular disease is more prevalent & accelerated with diabetes mellitus.

Risk factors

a. Hyper triglyceridemia (very low density lipo protein - VLDL)
b. Low levels of high density lipo protein (HDL)
c. Increase in cholesterol: Lecithin ratio

Pathogenesis: Enhanced non-enzymatic glycosylation of lipoprotein has been shown to impair the binding of glycosylated LDL to the LDL receptor. Glycosylated LDL enhances the formation of cholesteryl ester and accumulation of human macrophages - formation of foam cells characteristic of the early atheromatous lesion[7].
It is also noted that, vascular smooth muscle cells exhibit increased growth on exposure to high glucose in vitro.

Endothelium

Polyol pathway Advanced glycation products Diacyl glycerol Protein kinase pathway	} Proliferation[8] DNA damages Matrix protein synthesis Permeability Coagulation

Blue toe syndrome which is sudden onset of pain in the toe with bluish discoloration associated with leg/thigh myalgia and a sharp demarcated gangrenous toe is seen in diabetic foot. This is due to cholesterol emboli that break off from an ulcerated atheromatous plaque in the proximal vessels. Warfarin is used in treatment.
Microangiopathy: Hyperglycemia causes thickening of basement membrane of small vessels and capillaries due to incorporation of carbohydrates into basement membrane by induction of enzymes such as glycosyl, gactosyl transferase. Williamson et al observed that basement membrane thickening in the most dependent portion of the body may be the cause of increased hydrostatic pressure.
The chemical changes in basement membrane are:

- Increased hydroxylysine and glucose disaccharide content
- Decrease in proteoglycan and Heparin sulfate
- Increase in collagen type IV
- Decrease in lysine
- Decrease in laminin

Thickening interferes with transfer of oxygen and nutrients to the tissues and delays migration of leucocytes to the area of sepsis, there by delaying wound healing.
Haematological changes:
The haematological abnormalities are increased plasma and blood viscocity such as alteration in the plasma protein profile and disturbance in erythrocyte behavior. Erythrocytes are prone to increased aggregation and also show reduced deformability[10]. As glutathione metabolism is impaired in DM, the erythrocyte defenses against oxidative stress is impaired.
Haemostatic imbalances originate from acquired coagulation defects. The abnormalities of haemostatic system in DM are:

Endothelium	↓ Prostacyclin
	↓ Tissue factor production
Platelets:	↑ Hyper sensitivity to agonists
	↑ aggregation
	↓ Membrane fluidity
	↓ Platelet volume

Coagulation abnormalities are:
Coagulation factors

- ↑ Fibrinogen-
- ↑ factor VII, factor VIII and
- ↑ Von willebrands factor

Coagulation inhibitors

- ↓ Antithrombin III activity
- ↓ Heparin cofactor II activity
- ↓ Thrombin - antithrombin complex levels
- ↓ Protein C levels

Fibrinolysis abnormalities

- ↑ Plasminogen activator inhibitor
- Mega karyocyte platelet system is activated in diabetes mellitus.

Signs & symptoms of diabetic foot and leg caused by vascular abnormalities

1. Intermittent claudication
2. Cold feet
3. Rest pain
4. Absent pulses
5. Dependent rubour
6. Atrophic skin changes
7. Ulceration
8. Infection
9. Gangrene
   a. Type I patchy gangrene
   b. Type II extensive gangrene

3.3 Neuropathy in the diabetic foot

Peripheral neuropathies are found in 55% of diabetics. The incidence of neuropathies increases with duration of disease and episodes of neuropathies increases with duration of disease and episodes of hyperglycemia. Peripheral neuropathy clearly renders the patient to unrecognized injury, which potentates the risk of bacterial invasion and infection[11].

Definition of diabetic neuropathy: The presently accepted definition is demonstrable (clinical or sub clinical) disorder of somatic or autonomic parts of peripheral nervous system occurring in patients with DM[12]

Signs & symptoms

1. Paraesthesia
2. Hyperaesthesia
3. Hypoesthesia
4. Radicular pain
5. Loss of deep tendon reflexes
6. Loss of vibratory and position sense
7. Anhydrosis
8. Heavy callus formation over pressure points[13].
9. Infection complication of trophic ulcers
10. Foot drop

11. Change in bones and joints
12. Radiographic changes
    a. Demineralization
    b. Osteolysis
    c. Charcot joint

Aetiology

1. Vascular aetiology causing diabetic peripheral neuropathy[14].

Basement membrane thickening
Endothelial swelling & proliferation
Occlusive platelet thrombi
Closed capillaries

Multifocal ischaemic proximal nerve lesions[15].

Epineural vessel atherosclerosis
Decreased erythrocyte deformability

Nerve hypoxia

2. Metabolic Factors:

Accumulation of sorbitol
Decrease in nerve Na+ - K+ ATPase
Alteration in protein kinase C
Decrease in aminoacid incorporation into dorsal root ganglion.
Decrease in incorporation of glycolipids and amino acids into myelin
Excessive glycogen accumulation.
Nerve hypoxia

3. Other causes could be:

Increased nerve oedema
Increased blood nerve permeability
Decrease in endogenous nerve growth factor
Insulin deficiency.

3.4 Infections

In a normal individual the flora of the lower leg and foot are restricted because of following reasons:

1. Skin temperature is much lower than optimum for many human pathogens.
2. Metabolic products of skin have antimicrobial chemical effect.
3. Acid surface of the dorsum of foot & lower leg, making survival dependent on the ability of various microbes to resist drying.
4. Thick stratum corneum

Of all the infections seen in diabetic patient, bacterial and fungal infections of the skin are most common.

Predisposing factors:

a. Vascular insufficiency
b. Neuropathy.

Resistance to infection could be due to

a. Leukocyte mobilization.
b. Defective chemotaxis
c. Neutrophil bactericidal defects

Defect in formation of reactive oxygen metabolites[16].

Arterial insufficiency → locally tissues pressure & Metabolism

↓

Increased tissue demand for oxygen

↓

Increased extra vascular tension &
Local production of tissue destructive enzymes (phagocytes lysosomes)

↓

Local thrombosis and small vessel occlusion

↓

INFECTION

Commonest organisms are: Aerobes/Anaerobes

1. Gram negative bacilli : P. Mirabilis, E. Coli, P. Aeruginosa, E. Aerogenes
2. Gram – positive bacilli: Enterococcus Spp, S. Aureus, Group B. Strepto coccus

Anaerobes:

1. Gram negative bacilli: B. Fragilis, B. Ovatus, B. Ureolyticus
2. Gram positive bacilli: P.Magnus, P. Anaerobes, C. Bifirmentans

The infections are Polymicrobial in DM

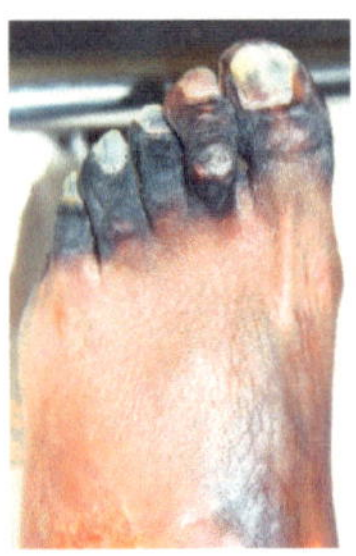

Dry gangrene

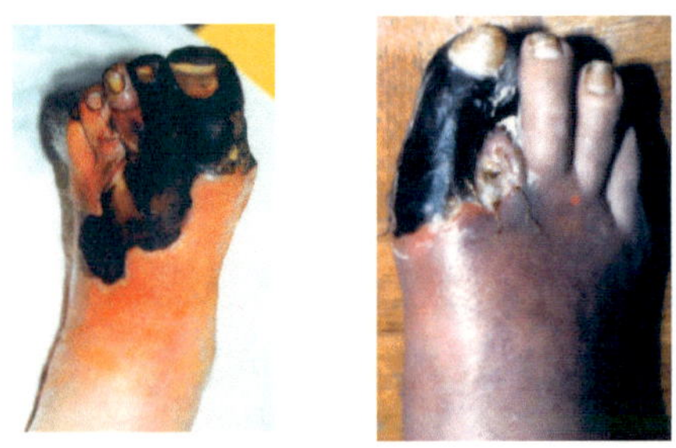

Wet gangrene

To summarise the pathogenesis, Salvapandian reviewed the different types of foot infections and their characteristics in 1982 [17]. These infections can occur in nondiabetic as well as diabetic persons, although the presence of the diabetic state can aggravate the risks and the morbidity associated with these infections. Post-traumatic foot infections can be classified as follows.

1. **Infected blister**: This is usually secondary to improperly fitting footwear, which causes separation of the superficial layers of the epidermis from the deeper layers.
2. **Infected abrasion**: This follows the traumatic removal of the horny layer of the skin, leaving the deeper layers open to the elements.
3. **Infected ulcer:** This usually is an extension of a previous abrasion and is usually due to pressure from the outside.
4. **Puncture wounds**
5. **Infected calluses**. These are usually a result of repeated intermittent pressure due to poorly fitting footwear and /or bony prominences and foot deformities as an end result of diabetic neuropathy and osteroarthropathy
6. **Infected corns**: These are conical wedges of keratinized tissue with the apices pointing inward. These usually occur on the heel or under metatarsal heads.

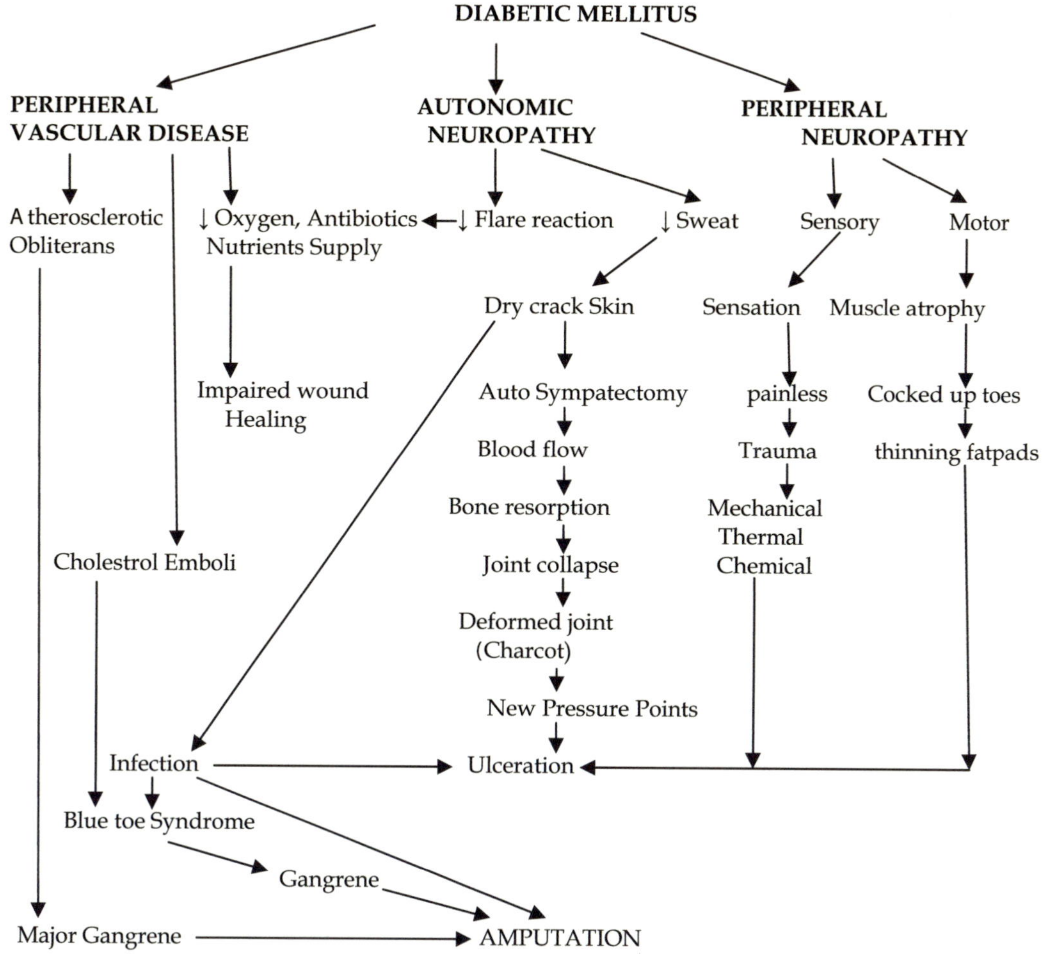

7. Infections following severe mechanical trauma such as in crush injuries or degloving injuries.
8. Infections can also follow the development of open areas in the skin such as the development of fissures. These fissures commonly occur between the toes or in the flexor creases of the toes.

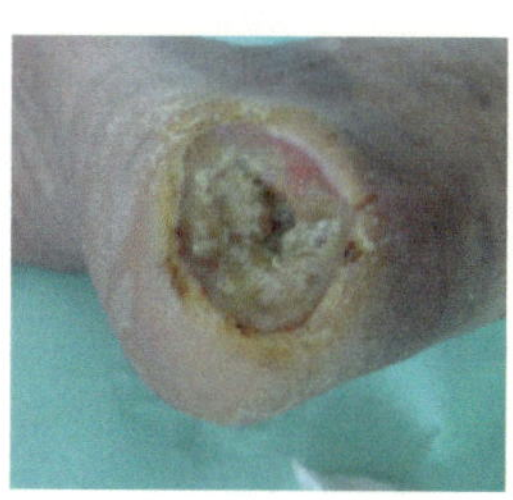
Infected ulcer in a diabetic patient

Depending on the severity of the illness and the extent of tissue involvement, these infections can vary in their clinical manifestations. Chronic poorly healing ulcers may be minimally symptomatic, but associated cellulites may result in fever, pain and tenderness in the involved area, and peripheral leukocytosis. The elderly diabetic patient may sometimes manifest no systemic symptoms.

Crepitant anaerobic cellulites is a disease entity that often results from mixed anaerobic and aerobic super infection of a long-standing diabetic foot ulcer. The infection gives rise to extensive gas formation that dissects underneath the skin, thus giving rise to crepitus on palpation. Patients usually demonstrate fever and leukocytosis. With appropriate management, this infection can usually be easily controlled.

Once pyogenic infections occur in the diabetic foot, they may ascend up the leg and sometimes progress to a necrotizing soft tissue infection. These infections are frequently caused by synergistic interaction of multiple bacteria, including anaerobes, aerobes, and microaerophilic bacteria. Included in these severe and life-threatening infections are synergistic necrotizing fasciitis and nonclostridial anaerobic myonecrosis (erstwhile erroneously called synergistic necrotizing cellulitis)[18].

4. Diabetic gangrene and vasculature

Atherosclerotic lesions in the arteries of diabetic patients occur at sites similar to those of non diabetic individuals (such as arterial bifurcations), while advanced disease is more common in diabetic patients, affecting even collateral vessels.

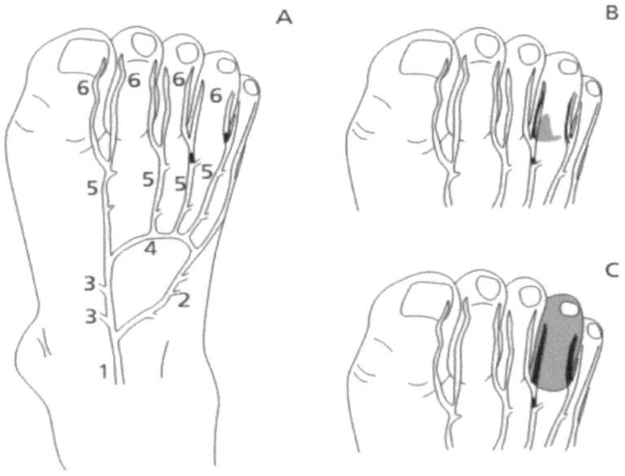

The pathology of the affected arteries is similar in both those with and those without diabetes. Typical atherosclerotic lesions in diabetic patients with peripheral vascular disease include diffuse multifocal stenosis and a predilection for the tibioperoneal arteries. All tibial arteries may be occluded, with distal reconstitution of a dorsal pedal or common plantar artery. Diabetes has the greatest impact on the smaller vessels (diameter less than 5 mm) in the body. The atherosclerotic procedure starts at a younger age and progresses more rapidly in those who have diabetics than those who do not. Although non - diabetic men are affected by peripheral vascular disease much more commonly than non- diabetic women (a male- to- female ratio of 30 : 1), diabetic women are affected half as often as diabetic men.

Gangrene is characterized by the presence of cyanotic, anesthetic tissue associated with or progressing to necrosis. It occurs when the arterial blood supply falls below minimal metabolic requirements. Gangrene can be described as dry or wet, wet gangrene being dry gangrene complicated by infection.

4.1 Blue toe syndrome

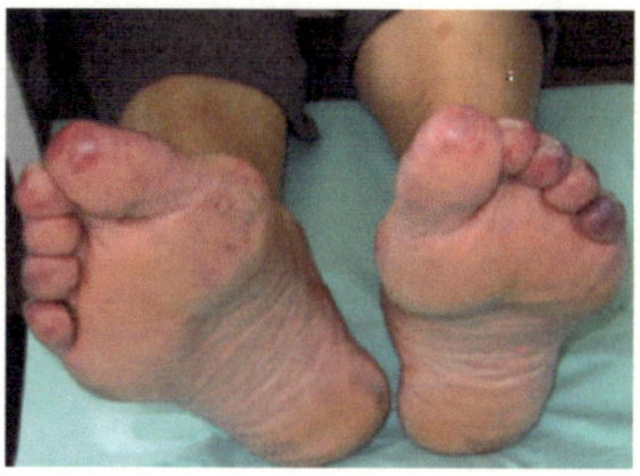

Ischemic purple patches on the toes and forefoot

4.2 Critical limb ischemia

Critical leg ischemia is any condition where there is an overwhelming likelihood that the limb is at risk for amputation or significant tissue loss within 6 months. The need for revascularization is more urgent than for patients with claudication. Critical limb ischemia occurs when distal limb perfusion is impaired to the extent that oxygen delivery is insufficient to meet resting metabolic tissue demands, and it follows inadequate adaptation of the peripheral circulation to chronic ischemia (collateral recruitment and vasodilatation). According to the consensus statement on critical limb ischemia (Norgren et al., 2007), critical leg ischemia is defined as either of the following two criteria:

a. persistently recurring ischemic rest pain requiring regular adequate analgesia for more than 2 weeks, with an ankle systolic pressure of 50 mmHg or less and/or a toe pressure of 30 mmHg or less;
b. ulceration or gangrene of the foot or toes, with an ankle systolic pressure of 50 mmHg or below and/or a toe pressure of 30 mmHg or less. In such patients, it is important to differentiate neuropathic pain from ischemic rest pain.

Critical leg ischemia is dominated by pedal pain (except in diabetic patients, where the superficial pain sensation may be altered and they may experience only deep ischemic pain, such as calf claudication and ischemic rest pain). In most cases, the pedal pain is intolerably severe; it may respond to foot dependency, but otherwise responds only to opiates.

Critical limb ischemia is manifested by rest pain (Rutherford classification category 4) or tissue loss. Rest pain is less frequent in individuals with diabetes because of the concomitant neuropathy. The rate of progression of peripheral arterial disease in patients with claudication to critical limb ischemia is 1.4% a year; progression is more likely in patients with diabetes and in tobacco smokers.

4.3 Diabetic gangrene ('end artery' disease)

In the normal foot, major injuries and operations are well tolerated by means of the arterial circulation distal to the ankle, since the plantar and the dorsal arches, their communications and the smaller arteries are patent. In the diabetic foot, however, smaller unnamed arteries may function as 'end - arteries ' due to multiple complete blockade and/or partial constrictive atherosclerotic lesions. Therefore local edema and thrombosis due to toxins produced by some bacteria (mainly staphylococci and streptococci) may cause ischemic necrosis of the tip of a toe or a part of its surface or of one or more toes, even when pulses are present in the foot arteries.

In the case of localized necrosis of the tip of a toe, removal of the gangrenous tissue, together with aggressive treatment of the infection, may lead to healing as long as the small arteries are still patent. Transluminal angioplasty or stenting of the occluded arteries will allow proper antibiotic treatment and salvage of the foot, while a gangrenous toe will be isolated by mummification (dry gangrene) without major consequences. Gangrene of the fifth toe or the hallux is due to more extended atherosclerotic disease and will probably lead to toe amputation or disarticulation.

4.4 Gangrene due to abscess of the plantar space

In a plantar space abscess, edema can obliterate the plantar arterial arch and its branches, leading to ischemia and necrosis of the middle toes, together with the central plantar space. The fifth toe and the hallux receive branches through the lateral and medial plantar spaces, respectively, and may survive central plantar space abscesses

4.5 Wet gangrene

A moist appearance, gross swelling and blistering characterize wet gangrene. Cellulitis (erythema) and the typical signs of inflammation are evident. Pus may be present. The patient may or may not be febrile, and pain is present unless there is loss of pain sensation due to diabetic neuropathy. Small vesicles or yellow, bluish or black bullae may form, and eventually a black eschar covers the infected necrotic area This is an emergency occurring in patients with severe ischemia who sustain an unrecognized trauma to their toe or foot. Urgent debridement of all affected tissues and the use of antibiotics often results in healing if sufficient viable tissue is present to maintain a functional foot, together with adequate circulation. If wet gangrene involves an extensive part of the foot, urgent guillotine amputation at a level proximal enough to encompass the necrosis and gross infection may be life - saving. At the same time, bypass surgery or a percutaneous transluminal angioplasty needs to be performed, if feasible. Saline gauze dressings, changed every 8 hours work well for open amputations. Revision to a below -knee amputation may be considered 3 – 5 days later. Wet gangrene is the most common cause of foot amputation in persons with diabetes. It often occurs in patients with severe peripheral vascular disease after infection. Dry gangrene may be infected and progress to wet gangrene.

Patients with dry gangrene who are awaiting a surgical procedure need education about meticulous foot care. It is extremely important for patients to avoid wet dressings and debriding agents, as their use may convert a localized dry gangrene to limb - threatening wet gangrene. Proper footwear is crucial to avoid further injury to the ischemic tissue.

4.6 Dry gangrene

Dry gangrene is characterized by its hard, dry and wrinkled dark brown or black texture; it usually occurs on the distal aspects of the toes often with a clear demarcation between viable and necrotic tissue. Once demarcation has occurs, the involved toes may be allowed to auto amputate. However, this process is long (several months) and disturbing. In addition, many patients do not have an adequate circulation to heal a distal amputation. For these reasons, it is common practice to evaluate the arteries angiographically and perform a bypass or a percutaneous transluminal angioplasty with concomitant limited distal amputation, in order to improve the chance of wound healing. In the case of extended gangrene, amputation at a higher level is unavoidable.

5. Lower Extremity Arterial Disease (LEAD)

The incidence and prevalence of LEAD increase with age in both diabetic and nondiabetic subjects and, in those with diabetes, increase with duration of diabetes. Many elderly diabetic persons have LEAD at the time of diabetes diagnosis. Diabetes is an important risk factor for LEAD. Hypertension, smoking, and hyperlipidemia, which are frequently present in patients with diabetes, contribute additional risk for vascular disease. LEAD in diabetes is compounded by the presence of peripheral neuropathy and by susceptibility to infection. These confounding factors in diabetic patients contribute to progression of LEAD to foot ulcerations, gangrene, and ultimately to amputation of part of the affected extremity. Prevention is an important component of LEAD management. By the time LEAD becomes clinically manifest, it may be too late to salvage an extremity, or it may require more costly resources to improve the circulatory health of the extremity.

LEAD manifests itself by decreased arterial perfusion to the lower extremities. This decreased perfusion results in diminution or absence of peripheral pulses and may lead to intermittent claudication (pain on walking, relieved promptly by rest), proneness to infection, ulcerations, poor healing of sores and ulcers, gangrene, and ultimately to amputation. Intermittent claudication is indicative of clinical occlusive LEAD.

Palpation of peripheral pulses has been used as a clinical tool to assess occlusive LEAD in diabetic and nondiabetic patients, particularly when intermittent claudication is present. However, it is sometimes difficult to interpret the significance of diminished peripheral pulses when symptoms are not present. Ambient temperature, anatomic variation, and expertise in palpating peripheral pulses may contribute to variation in the clinical examination. Absence of pulses remains a significant clinical finding. Absent posterior tibial, popliteal, or femoral pulses with or without bruits that persist on repeated examination are clinically significant and indicate significant occlusive LEAD whether intermittent claudication is present or not.

Angiography remains the gold standard for identifying occlusive LEAD and the areas of occlusion in the arterial system. Patients being considered for amputation because of occlusive LEAD should have angiography performed to determine whether revascularization may be effective in salvaging the limb or in lowering the level of amputation.

Diabetic vasculature

Two types of vascular disease are seen in patients with diabetes: a **non occlusive micro circulatory dysfunction** involving the capillaries and arterioles of the kidneys, retina, and peripheral nerves, and a **macroangiopathy** characterized by atherosclerotic lesions of the coronary and peripheral arterial circulation. The former is relatively unique to diabetes, whereas the latter lesions are morphologically and functionally similar in both non diabetic and diabetic patients. As it became increasingly evident that the vasculature of the foot was spared the changes noted in the more proximal vessels, measurement of digital toe pressures was initiated. Subsequent study has confirmed that toe pressures are not hampered by the coexistence of diabetes. In fact, Vincent et al. showed that toe pressure was an accurate hemodynamic indicator of total peripheral arterial obstructive disease in diabetics.

Angiography is indicated in the diabetic patients with non healing ulcers or osteomyelitis requiring endovascular and surgical planning. Almost without exception, these patients with nonhealing foot ulcers will have severe stenoocclusive disease involving all three runoff vessels of the calf (anterior tibial, posterior tibial, and peroneal arteries). In this patient population, 20% of peripheral bypass grafts will have to extend to a pedal artery. The distal anastomosis is either to the dorsalis pedis artery or the proximal common plantar artery trunk (54). Thus detailed mapping of arterial disease from the abdominal aorta to the pedal vessels is necessary. Besides palpation and bedside Doppler evaluation of pulses, the clinical examination should include a standard assessment of skin color, turgor, and temperature. Edema may be present, which thwarts a thorough physical examination of pulses. A "Dopplered" pedal pulse should be at least biphasic, to support healing. If there is any doubt about the adequacy of perfusion, then noninvasive studies should be obtained. The ankle-brachial index (ABI) may be unreliable in patients with noncompressible lower-leg vessels. In general, however, an ABI of less than 0.5 in the setting of a nonhealing wound indicates a need for vascular reconstruction. According to Colen and Musson, an ABI of 0.7 or greater is appropriate if a free flap with a distal arterial anastomosis is planned.

Gangrene

Gangrene is defined as focal or extensive necrosis of the skin and underlying tissue. However, this definition presents difficulties. There are several etiologies for gangrene, as there are for foot ulcers. One is LEAD of the large or small vessels, but infection and neuropathy may also play a role. Gangrene is better correlated with LEAD than is foot ulcer. The demonstration of clinical or subclinical LEAD is essential if gangrene is to be considered a manifestation of the progression of LEAD in the individual patient. The prevalence of gangrene is greater in selected diabetic patient populations than in the general community. However, prevalence is not a satisfactory indicator of the importance of gangrene in diabetes, compared with incidence, because of the poor survival experience of these patients and their consequent loss from the prevalent population. Risk factors for gangrene have not been adequately quantified for diabetic patients. They include LEAD, peripheral neuropathy, infection, trauma, and delayed healing.

6. Investigations

The initial assessment of PAD in patients with diabetes should begin with a thorough medical history and physical examination to help identify those patients with PAD risk factors, symptoms of claudication, rest pain, and/or functional impairment. Alternative causes of leg pain on exercise should be excluded. PAD patients present along a spectrum of severity ranging from no symptoms, intermittent claudication, rest pain, and finally to nonhealing wounds and gangrene.

Palpation of peripheral pulses should be a routine component of the physical exam and should include assessment of the femoral, popliteal, and pedal vessels. It should be noted that pulse assessment is a learned skill and has a high degree of interobserver variability, with high false-positive and false-negative rates. The dorsalis pedis pulse is reported to be absent in 8.1% of healthy individuals, and the posterior tibial pulse is absent in 2.0%. Nevertheless, the absence of both pedal pulses, when assessed by a person experienced in this technique, strongly suggests the presence of vascular disease.

The ABI is measured by placing the patient in a supine position for 5 min. Systolic blood pressure is measured in both arms, and the higher value is used as the denominator of the ABI. Systolic blood pressure is then measured in the dorsalis pedis and posterior tibial arteries by placing the cuff just above the ankle. The higher value is the numerator of the ABI in each limb.

The diagnostic criteria for Peripheral artery disease (PAD) based on the ABI are interpreted as follows:

Normal if 0.91–1.30
Mild obstruction if 0.70–0.90
Moderate obstruction if 0.40–0.69
Severe obstruction if <0.40
Poorly compressible if >1.30

An ABI value >1.3 suggests poorly compressible arteries at the ankle level due to the presence of medial arterial calcification. This makes the diagnosis by ABI alone less reliable.
The following investigations are done for the diagnosis and treatment of diabetic foot:

1. To demonstrate the extent and severity of the disease process.
2. To screen diabetic patients for peripheral vascular insufficiency.
3. To confirm and control the intercurrent diseases interfering with the healing process.

6.1 Urine examination

- Albumin
- Sugar

6.2 Culture and sensitivity tests

Pus from infected area is cultured for microorganisms and their sensitivity to various antibiotics.

6.3 X-Ray

X-ray of the foot should be taken to rule out osteomyelitis. The sign, which suggests the presence of osteomyelitis, is destruction of bone commonly seen at metatarsophalangeal joint or in the interphalangeal joint of the great toe. Sequestrum and subperiosteal new bones formations are common. A small amount of gas in the tissues or in the abscess cavity may be seen. Large amounts of subcutaneous gas indicates the presence of a serious anaerobic infection. In severe ischaemia, there may be generalised osteoporosis in the bone of the foot.

6.4 Non-invasive evaluation

The non-invasive techniques assumed an important role in peripheral arterial ischaemic diseases. They give an accurate assessment of anatomic and physiologic vascular status

a. **Toe pressure** They provide a highly accurate method for determining the success in the healing of an ulcer or in minor amputation. A toe pressure of 20 - 30 mm Hg below which healing is doubtful.
b. **Duplex scanning with ultrasound analysis (doppler study)** The recorded Doppler signal is used in two ways:
   - To measure segmental systolic pressure
   - To provide flow velocity wave form patterns for analysis.

   Colour Doppler scanners Colour Doppler scanners detect and display moving structures by superimposing colour onto the grey-scale image. The hue of the colour can be used to identify sites where the artery becomes narrower and the blood has to move faster to achieve the same volume flow rate.

c. **Others**
- Photoplethysmography
- Segmental pressure
- Waveform evaluation

6.5 Invasive techniques

a. Angiography

Percutaneous femoral angiography

Anatomic evaluation of the vascular supply to the leg and foot require arteriography. In young patients with vascular insufficiency diagnosis of obstruction can be made when arteriogram show severe diffuse atherosclerotic disease involving the tibial and peroneal arteries. The possibility of large vessel stenosis are occlusion superimposing on distal possibility of large vessel stenosis are occlusion superimposing on distal diabetic vascular disease is most important indication for angiography.

b. Digital subtraction angiography

The term digital subtraction angiography refers to visualization of vessels using digital fluoroscopic techniques for image enhancement.

c. Radionuclide bone scintigraphy:
- Bone scanning using technetium 99m phosphonates is useful in identifying early osteomyelitis.
- Gallium accumulates in areas of active inflammation
- Sequential gallium scan are useful in monitoring the response to treatment for chronic osteomyelitis.

d. Computed tomography
- Well suited for imaging complex articulations and numerous soft tissue structure.
- Can identify and characterize the extent of soft tissue infection.

e. Magnetic resonance imaging
- Detects and displays bone marrow alterations in osteomyelitis
- Displays the contrast between soft tissue, medullary tissue and cortex with clarity.

7. Prognosticating factors

Chance of Ischemic Rest Pain Ankle pressure	Unlikely	Probable	Likely
Non diabetic	More than 55	35 - 55	Less than 35
Diabetic	More than 80	55-80	Less than 55

Prediction of Healing of Ulcer Ankle pressure	Likely	Probable	Unlikely
Non diabetic	More than 65	55 - 65	Less than 55
Diabetic	More than 90	80 - 90	Less than 80

Chance of below knee Amputation Healing Diabetics	Likely	Probable	Unlikely
Calf pressure	More than 65	More than 65	Less than 65
Ankle pressure	More than 30	More than 30	Less than 30

CHART FOR MANAGEMENT OF DIABETIC FOOT

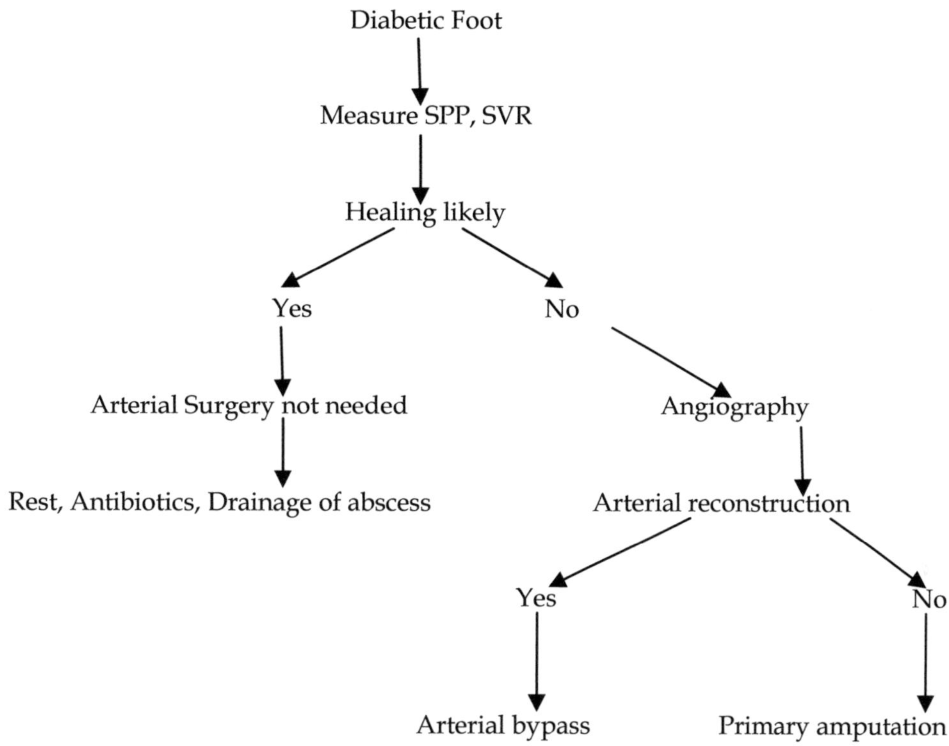

8. Management of diabetic gangrene

The management of diabetic gangrene has to be individualized. Factors that have to be considered include manifestations of sepsis, the extent of tissue necrosis and gangrene, the adequacy of the vascularity to the involved limb, the extent and severity of the soft tissue infection, the presence and extent of bone involvement, the severity of the peripheral neuropathy, the presence and severity of foot deformity, and the metabolic control of the diabetic state. If the diabetes is not adequately controlled, insulin therapy should be initiated.
Surgical intervention is of paramount importance in most of these infections. Some patients may benefit from vascular reconstruction, since patients with nonhealing or poorly healing ulcers secondary to vascular insufficiency may heal following vascular surgery.

8.1 Antimicrobial therapy

Mild infections: If there are no clinical manifestations of sepsis, mono antibiotic therapy may be instituted while awaiting culture and sensitivity reports. In the absence of necrotic tissue, foul smelling discharge & frank gangrene, it is more common to isolate single microorganisms and anaerobes are relatively uncommon[19]. In this, gram +ve aerobic cocci are usually dominant organisms.
Included under these: Staphylococcus aureus, Coagulase –ve staphylococci, Nongroup D streptococci, Entercocci
First generation Cepholosporins will cover first 2 organisms, but are inactive against remaining organisms. Ticarcillin - Clavulanate and imipenem will be adequate for most

coagulase positive and negative staphylococci. For Gram +ve organisms Ampicillin - Sulbactum will provide adequate coverage.

Severe infections: In the presence of more severe infections, especially when tissue necrosis and gangrene are present, when the infections process is rapidly progressive and / or when toxaemia, hypotensive shock, and other signs of sepsis are present, more broad spectrum, antibiotic therapy is indicated. In addition to staphylococci and entercococci, anaerobes as B fragilis and gram -ve aerobic bacilli P. aeruginosa are frequently isolated and may respond to clindamycin[20].

Metronidazole is excellent against Gram-negative anaerobic bacilli, but has limited activity against gram positive anaerobic and microaerophilic cocci. Imipenem, ticarcillin clavulanate and ampicillin - sulbactum all have excellent activity against almost all anaerobic bacteria[21]

There is reluctance in using amino glycosides in diabetic patients due to evidence of diabetic nephropathy in these patients and amino glycosides might worsen the nephropathy[22]. The choice of an antipseudomonal agent is likely to be antipseudomonal B- lactam or quinolines. With severe infections or presence of toxaemia or septicemia, it may be prudent to use a combination of atleast two antimicrobial agents as preliminary empirial therapy pending knowledge of deep tissue culture & sensitivity.

8.2 Saving the diabetic foot

One of the primary goals of treating diabetes is to save the diabetic foot. This can be achieved by

1. Correction of vascular risk factors
2. Improved circulation
3. Proper treatment of diabetic foot ulcers
4. Team work
5. Patient education in foot care

CORRECTION OF VASCULAR RISK FACTORS.

Risk factors for micro vascular disease are given in table below. Certain risk factors can be controlled and hence should be.

Risk factors for micro vascular disease

Non treatable	Treatable	Miscellaneous
Genetic	Smoking	Inotropic drugs
Age	Hypertension	Beta blockers
Diabetes	Hypercholestrolemia	
Duration of diabetes	Hypertriglyceridemia	
	Hypoglycemia	

Hyperinsulinemia may lead to increased atherosclerosis. First it can induce deposition of fat into the macrophages or foam cells that part of stenotic plaque. Insulin also by growth hormone like action stimulates mitotic division and growth of smooth muscle cells from media into plaque.

IMPROVED CIRCULATION

Exercise is important in building up collaterals. Vasodilators have a very minimal role, as diabetes is not a vasospastic condition. Antiplatelet drugs like aspirin and dispyridamole can be used. The basic pathology in blood is hypercoagulability and change in rheologic properties of RBC. The ability of the RBC to change shape is lost to certain degree.

Pentoxyphylline is a drug, which can increases the red cell flexibility. Thus blood flow can be increased and blood viscosity decreased.

9. Wagner's grading of foot lesions

Wagner (1983) grades lesions of diabetic foot from 0-5 by depth and extent.
Grade 0 No ulcer but high risk foot
Grade 1 Superficial ulcer (commonest site is head of 1st metatarsal).
Grade 2 Deep ulcer with no bony involvement
Grade 3 Abscess with bony involvement
Grade 4 Localised gangrene
Grade 5 Gangrene of whole foot
GRADE 0 FEET
No open lesions but is an at risk foot.
A large amount of callus under a metatarsal head may act as a foreign body and lead to ulcer in an open but hidden lesion and if present should be reclassified as Grade1.
Grade 0 feet with deformities such as intrinsic, minus, hammer or claw toes, charcot's joint or hallux valgus need purpose designed shoes. Proper patient education plays a key role in the management of diabetic patients with Grade 0 feet.
GRADE 01 LESION
Superficial ulcer but with thickness skin loss. Usually these occur in plantar surfaces of toes of metatarsal heads. But "Kission lesion" occurs in between toes caused by over-tight shoes. This is due to repeated pressure leading to ischemia. Thus mainstay of treatment is to release pressure from ulcerated area, surrounding callus removal and ulcer debridement until healthy granulation is seen. Saline irrigation is usually enough in these relatively clean superficial ulcers. If infection is present, a wound swab should be taken and antibiotic therapy with broad-spectrum agents should be started immediately. The most important part of treatment is to relieve pressure till lesions heal.
GRADE 02 LESIONS
Ulcer is deep and often penetrates subcutaneous fat down to tendon or ligament, but without abscess or bony infection. These patients should be admitted to hospital and blood and ulcer cultures should be taken and foot X-rayed.
Culture for aerobes and anaerobes should be done. Staphylococci and bacteroides are one of the two commonest isolates. Fluocloxacillin and Metronidazole are used as blind first line therapy. Deep infected ulcer need to be debrided either in ward or under general anesthesia. After debridement, deep ulcer should be packed with Eusol and paraffin in 175 mm or 250 mm gauze wick to encourage healthy granulation tissue growth. Otherwise simple dry dressing is advised. Topical antibiotics are not useful.
GRADE 03 LESIONS
Deep infection with cellulitis or abscess formation often with underlying osteomyelities. In management, surgery is often needed. Foot X-ray ulcer and blood cultures is a must.
Absent foot pulses, low ankle pressure and diffuse arterial disease suggest that lesion will not heal without amputation. If available Doppler studies may help to decide whether to persist with conservative treatment or proceed with local amputation. If the lesion is purely neuropathic, conservative treatment is sufficient since ulcer usually heals. Initial treatment constitutes bed rest, elevation of foot, antibiotics according to culture and sensitivity. Optimal glycaemic control is also needed. Grade 3 foot with good blood supply can often be

treatment with amputation, with surgical drainage, dressing and wound irrigation. Amputation may be needed if severe infection or progressive anaerobic infection is present.

GRADE 04 LESIONS

Treatment is same as Grade 3 lesion. Avoid pressure bearing either with special shoes or bed rest is the mainstay of treatment. When distal vascularity is adequate it is worthwhile trying conservatism. Arteriography is indicated to see whether bypass or angioplasty is indicated. If neither is possible, if there is no rest pain, then a period of conservative treatment is worthwhile. A painless black toe with dry gangrene often amputates spontaneously if left alone. In a previously mobility patient, a below knee amputation is better than above knee amputation because of better rehabilitation.

GRADE 05 LESIONS

These patients have extensive gangrene of the foot and needs urgent hospital admission, control of diabetes and infection and major amputation.

10. Buerger's disease (thromboangittis obliterans)[23]

Characterized in histology by thrombosis in both arteries and veins with marked inflammatory reaction. This classic condition described by Buerger involves young men with severe ischaemia of the extremities who are addicted to cigarette smoking and often have migratory superficial phlebitis.

Definition - It is an inflammatory reaction in the arterial wall with involvement of the neighbouring vein and nerve, terminating in thromboses of the artery. It is probably presenile atherosclerosis occurring in the 3rd, 4th,and 5th decades of the life.

Incidence - more frequently in men between 20 and 40 years of age. It is uncommon in women, who constitute only 5% to 10% of all patients with Buerger's disease.

Aetiology - interaction of multiple aetiologic factors. There is striking association of this disease with **cigarette smoking.** (> 20 cigarettes per day) There may be some **hormonal influence** which suggests the sex distribution. Patients often come from **lower socio-economic groups**. A **hypercoagulable state** has been postulated. There has also been report of hyperaggregability of platelets. **Familial predisposition** has been reported. **Autonomic overactivity** has been suggested by a few pathologists, as there is also sometimes peripheral vasospasm and hyperhidrosis noticed in this condition. Recently an **autoimmune aetiology** has been postulated.

Pathology - An obvious inflammatory process features the Buerger's disease involving all layers of the vessel wall. Thrombus is noticed in the lumen of the affected artery. There are also microabscesses within the thrombus. In the late stage the affected artery becomes occluded and contracted with marked fibrotic reaction affecting all the layers of the artery e.g. the adventitia, the media and intima. This fibrotic process gradually involves the vein and adjacent nerves. The lesions in Buerger's disease are segmental and usually begin in arteries of small and medium size. Both upper and lower extremities are affected.

Clinical features. It is characterized as peripheral ischaemia, particularly if the upper extremity is involved and it there is a history of migratory superficial phlebitis.

SYMPTOMS Complain of pain at the arch of the foot (foot claudication) while walking. Pain is typical of intermittent claudication type. Intermittent claudication progresses to rest pain. Gradually postural colour changes appear followed by trophic changes, eventually ulceration and gangrene of one or more digits and finally of the entire foot or hand may take place. When rest pain develops, it is so intense that the patient cannot sleep. If the affected limb is kept in dependent position some relief of pain may be obtained. The limbs become rubor or red on dependence and pallor on elevation.

Special Investigations: Arteriography is the most important investigation in this condition. In arteriography it is the peripheral arteries which are first involved There is usually extensive collateral circulation surrounding the involved arteries which look like 'tree-roots' or 'spider legs'. In approximately 1/4th of cases one can find a characteristic 'cork-screw' appearance in the vicinity of the affected artery, presumably due to greatly dilated vasa vasorum of the occluded artery

Treatment - Pain is the most important symptom of Buerger's disease which requires to be relieved. Narcotics may be necessary, but one must be careful against drug addiction.

CONSERVATIVE TREATMENT has a great role to play -

1. Stop smoking.
2. Various drugs have been tried with different degrees of success. Vasodilator drugs, anticoagulants, dextran, phenylbutazone, inositol and steroids have all been tried. More recently prostaglandin therapy (PGA-1) has been advocated to prevent platelet aggregation.

SURGICAL TREATMENT -

1. Role of sympathectomy is doubtful.
2. Arterial reconstruction is also difficult
3. Free omental graft for revascularisation of ischaemic extremity
4. Amputation is the only way out when gangrene occurs. The approach is conservative and lowest possible level should be chosen.

Prognosis - The risk of amputation is about 20% within 10 years after onset of symptoms. Although this varies with the use of tobacco. In a few patients who stop smoking completely, progression of the disease is greatly restricted.

11. Osteomyelitis in diabetic patients[24,25,26]

Osteomyelitis is difficult to cure, even in normal bone, because of bone's limited blood flow. An infection in bone results when bacteria are able to colonize ischemic or injured areas where the blood supply is not adequate to combat the infection with its normal defenses. As bacteria grow in this ischemic bone, they cause further bone death by vessel injury from decreases in pH, oxygen, and nutrients and increases in pressure and metabolites. When bone's blood supply is further limited by diabetic vasculitis and then by osteomylitis, cure is more difficult. The oxygen tension of infected bone in the diabetic patient is about one-quarter that of the overlying soft tissue, which may also be very low. This ischemia is accompanied by metabolic and pH changes that decrease or prevent normal immunologic defenses and antibiotic penetrance and efficacy, and increase bacterial growth. Furthermore, the diabetic individual has decreased phagocytosis by polymorph nuclear leukocytes and decreased T-cell function. These factors make diabetic osteomyelitis a challenge to treat.

STAGES OF OSTEOMYELITIS

Stage I - infection is simple with no permanent anatomic damage. This is medullary osteomyelitis in a bone, acute septic arthritis in a joint, or cellulitis of soft tissue.

Stage II- is superficial periosteal or cortical osteomyelitis, chondrolysis, sub-acute septic remains arthritis, or ulcerated soft tissue.

Stage III- the infection is deeper but localized. It involves both the cortex and the medullary canal for osteomyelitis, bone about the joint for septic arthritis, or an abscess in soft tissue.

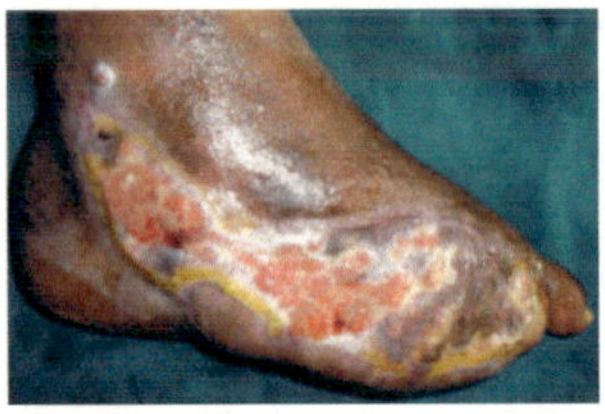

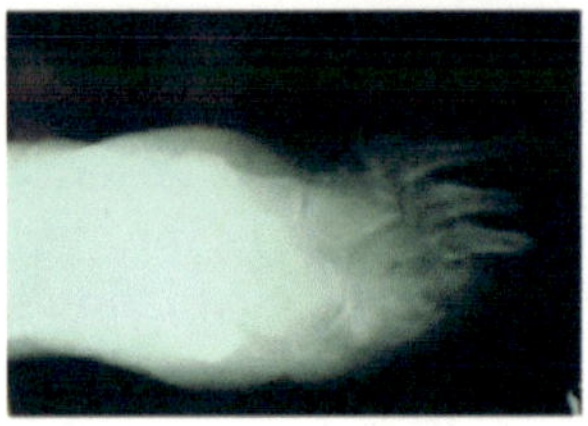

Stage IV- infection is diffuse, diffuse osteomyelitis (nonunion), end stage septic arthritis (unstable joint), or a permeating necrotizing infection (gas gangrene, necrotizing fasciitis)
Treatment Goals There are three possible treatment goals for diabetic osteomyelitis:
ARREST: "Arresting" osteomyelitis, means to debride the infection to the subthreshold level of bacteria so local tissue and antibiotics can heal the wound. Unfortunately, this is difficult for diabetic patients because of rapidly progressing ischemia.
SUPPRESSION: Suppressive therapy requires the highest amount of patient compliance and physician clinical time. An open wound is debrided in the clinic. Local wound care is done at home, and suppressive antibiotics are used to control cellutitis or progression of infection. Suppressive antibiotics are used to control cellulitis or progression of infection.
AMPUTATIONS: The team consists of a vascular surgeon, an orthopedic surgeon, and a physiotherapist and rehabilitation expert.

12. Determination of the level of amputation

Level of amputation is determined by the site at which wound healing will occur easily and leads to a residual limb which can be functionally useful. Unfortunately in diabetic patients, occlusive vascular disease leading to diabetic foot is often bilateral. That means 30-40% of such people will require amputation of the opposite limb within 2-3 years.
Many clinical signs suggest level of amputation like skin changes, vascular pulsation, and peripheral neuropathy and rest pain.
It is found that 70 mm arterial pulse at desired amputation level or a leg to arm pressure ratio more than or equal to 0.45 was found to be satisfactory and statistically valid in 80-90% patients. Occasionally patients with arterial calcification and inelastic vessel walls show abnormally high blood pressure. But waveform evaluation detects the problem. Final decision regarding level of amputation is taken as late as putting the skin incision. **SURGICAL TECHNIQUE** The gangrenous foot or leg is covered with a plastic bag or drape. Remainder of exposed limb is thoroughly cleaned with 10-minute surgical wash followed by povidone iodine solution.

12.1 Amputation of toes

- Amputation of terminal phalanx of great toe

For a functionally useful stump it is important to preserve the base of terminal phalanx

- Amputation through proximal phalanx of great toe

Not more than the base of phalanx should be therefore preserved.

- Amputation of great toe at its base

12.2 Disarticulation of the metatarsophalyngeal joints

- Disarticulations of lateral four toes: Racquet approach is employed.
- **Amputation of all other toes**: Toes are disarticulated at the metatarsophalangeal joint

12.3 Amputation of foot

- **Transmetatarsal amputations** This amputation is undertaken using a long posterior flap, which extend to a level just proximal to the flexion crease at the base of toes.
- **Tarsometatarsal amputation (Lisfrank level)** This is performed through the tarsometatarsal joints and usually results in good partial amputations.
- **Midtarsal amputation (Chopart amputation)** It is a disarticulation between the oscalcis and cuboid bones and talus and navicular bones and is seldom used.
- **Syme's amputation** The tibia and fibula are divided at or immediately above the level of ankle joint. The ends are covered with a single flap obtained from skin of heel.
- **Modified syme's amputation** this modification has nothing to commend and hence not widely approved.

12.4 Below knee amputation

Amputation at the below knee level through middle 3rd of leg is the operation of choice when it is not possible to conserve the foot and heel. Ideal length of tibial stump is 14 cm.

12.5 Above knee amputation

Patient can be fitted with preparatory lower limb prosthesis approximately 3-4 weeks after operation depending on healing of wound. Definitive prosthesis is usually put after 2-4 months.

13. References

[1] Kumar Kamal, Richard JP, Bauer ES. The pathology of diabetes mellitus, implication for surgeons. Journal of American College of Surgeons. 1996 Septembger; 183:271.

[2] Gayle R, Benjamin AL, Gary NG. The burden of diabetic foot ulcers. The American Journal of Surgery 1998Aug 24; 176(Suppl 2A):65-105.

[3] Britlan ST, Young RJ, Sharma AK, Clarks BF. Relationship of endonetal capillary abnormalities to type and severity of diabetic polyneuropathy. Diabetes 1990; 39:909-913

[4] Farad JV, Sotalo J. Low serum levels of nerve growth factor in diabetic neuropathy. Acta Neurol Scand 1990; 81:402-406

[5] Viswanathan V. Profile of diabetic foot complications and its associated complications – a multicentric study from India. Journal of Association of Physicians of India 2005 Nov; 53:933-6

[6] Pyorala K, Laasko M, Vusiitupa M. Diabetes and atherosclerosis, An epidemiologic view. Diabet Methob Rev 1987; 3:463-524

[7] Lopes Verella MF, Klein RH, Lyon TJ. Glycosylation of low density lipoprotein enhance cholesteryl ester synthesis in human monocyte derived macdrophage diabgetes 1988; 37:550-557

[8] Natarajan R, Gonzalez N, XVI, NEdler JL. Vascular smooth muscle cell exhibit increased growth in response to elevated glucose. Biochem Biophys Res Commun 1992; 187:552-560

[9] Tooke JE. Microvascular hemodynamics in diabetes mellitus. Clin Sci 1986; 70:119-125

[10] Mac Rury SM, Lowe GDO. Blood rheology in DM. Diabet Med 1990; 7:285-291

[11] Edmol ME. Experience in a multi disciplinary diabetic foot clinic. In The foot in diabetes, Cornor H, Boulton AJM, Wards JD (eds). 1st edition. Chichester, England: John Wiley and Sons Ltd 1987; 121-134
[12] Harati Y. Frequently asked questions about diabetic peripheral neuropathies. Neurologic Clinic 1992 Aug; 10(3):783-801
[13] Delbring L, Ctectelco G, Fowler C. The etiology of diabetic neuropathic ulceration. Br J Surgery 1985; 72:1-6
[14] Britlan ST, Young RJ, Sharma AK, Clarks BF. Relationship of endonetal capillary abnormalities to type and severity of diabetic polyneuropathy. Diabetes 1990; 39:909-913
[15] Sugimura K, Duck PJ. Multifonal fibre loss in proximal sciatic nerve in symmetrical distal diabetic neuropathy. Neurol Sci 1982; 53:501
[16] Shah SV, Wallen JD, Eilen SD. Chemiluminescene and superoxide anion production by leukocyte from diabetic patients. J Clin Endocrinol Metab 1983
[17] Salvapandian AJ. Infections of the foot. In: Disorders of the foot, Iahss MH (ed). Philadelphia: WB Saunders 1982; 401
[18] Bessman AN, Sapico FL, Tobatabai MF, Montgomerie JZ. Persistence of polymicrobial abscesses in poorly controlled diabetic host. Diabetes 1986; 36:448
[19] Leslie CA, Sapico FL, Ginunas VJ, Adkins RH. Randomized clinical trial of tropical hyperbaric oxygen for treatment of diabetic foot ulcers. Diabetes Care 1988; 11:111
[20] Curchural GJ JR, Tally FP, Jacobus NV. Susceptibility of the bacteroids fragilis
[21] Rolfe RD, Finegold SM. Comparative in vitro activity of new beta-lactum antibiotics against anaerobic bacteria. Antimicrob Ag Chemother 1981; 20:600
[22] Moore RD, Smith CR, Lipsky JJ. Risk factors for nephrotoxicity in patient treated with aminoglycosides. Ann Internal Medicine 1984; 100:352
[23] Short cases of surgery by Das, India
[24] Van Dan Brands P, Welch W. Diagnosis of arterial occlusive disease of the lower extremities by laser flow Doppler flowmetry. Inter Angio 1988; 7:224
[25] Oberg PA, Tenland Nilsson GE. Laser Doppler flowmetry on non-invasive and microvascular and cautious method of blood flow evaluation in microvascular studies. Acta Med Scand Supp 1983; 17:687
[26] Matsen FA, Wyss CR, Robertson CL. The relationship of transcutaneous PO2 and Laser Doppler measurements in a human model of local arterial insufficiency. Surgery Gynaecology, Obstetrics 1984; 159, 148
[27] Atlas of diabetic foot, second edition, wiley-blackwell publications, 2010.

Part 4

Necrosis and Gangrene: Current Management Options

12

Effect of Macrolide Antibiotics on Biological Activities Induced by *Clostridium perfringens* Alpha-Toxin

Jun Sakurai and Masataka Oda
Faculty of Pharmaceutical Sciences, Tokushima Bunri University
Japan

1. Introduction

Clostridium perfringens type A (*C. perfringens*) causes gas gangrene with inflammatory myopathies and infrequently septicemia associated with massive intravascular hemolysis. The gas gangrene involves any part of the body; the most common sites being the toes, fingers, feet, and hands. Features include localized pain, swelling and myonecrosis, and finally, shock and death. The septicemia with massive hemolysis and fever leads to death within a few hours.

The microorganism is known to produce a variety of toxins and enzymes that are responsible for severe myonecrotic lesions. Notably, alpha-toxin, which possesses hemolytic, necrotic and lethal activities, and phospholipase C (PLC) and sphingomyelinase (SMase) activities, is an important agent for the diseases (Bryant et al. 2000, Sakurai, Nagahama and Oda 2004). It has been reported that the toxin is required for myonecrosis, hemolysis, inhibition of neutrophil infiltration and thrombosis (Stevens and Bryant 1997, Awad et al. 2001, Ellemor et al. 1999). We also reported that the toxin stimulated O_2^- production in neutrophils, and firm adhesion of the cells to matrix ligands, fibrinogen, fibronectin, and collagen (Ochi et al. 2002), suggesting that the toxin stimulates the binding of neutrophils to the vascular endothelium and inflammation there. The findings suggest that neutrophils activated by the toxin are unable to migrate across the vascular endothelium in an infectious focus. Actually, gas gangrene caused by *C. perfringens* is reported to be a fulminant necrotizing infection in which inflammatory cells are notably absent from infected tissues, but are often accumulated in vascular wall (Bunting et al. 1997).

Stevens et al. reported that alpha-toxin may cause shock indirectly by stimulating the release of endogenous mediators (Bryant and Stevens 1996, Stevens 2000). We found that the intravenous injection of alpha-toxin in mice resulted in the release of various cytokines (Oda et al. 2008). Cytokines are immunoregulatory peptides with a strong inflammatory action, mediating the immune/metabolic response to an external noxious stimulus and later the transition from septicemia to septic shock, multiple organ dysfunction syndromes, and/or multiple organ failure (Tracey et al. 1987, Riedemann, Guo and Ward 2003, Dinarello 2004). It is thought that synergistic interactions between cytokines can cause or attenuate tissue injury (Calandra, Bochud and Heumann 2002). Tumor necrosis factor (TNF)-α, released from neutrophils, macrophages, and endothelial cells, is an important cytokine involved in the pathophysiology of septicemia (Tracey et al. 1987, Lum et al. 1999). TNF- α-induced tissue injury is largely mediated through neutrophils which respond by producing elastase, superoxide ion, hydrogen peroxide, phospholipase A, platelet-activating factor, leukotriene B1, and thromboxane A2 (Aldridge 2002). Therefore, it is possible that the exacerbation of gas gangrene with inflammatory symptom and septicemia with massive intravascular hemolysis caused by *C. perfringens* is dependent on cytokines released from neutrophils and macrophages activated by the toxin.

Macrolide antibiotics, including erythromycin (ERM), azithromycin (AZM), clarithromycin and kitasamycin (KTM), are recognized as potent antibiotics for the treatment of various microbial infections (Schmid 1971). Some of these antibiotics have been reported to be effective against diffuse panbronchiolitis characterized by chronic inflammation with inflammatory cell infiltration (Kadota et al. 1993, Fujii et al. 1995). Thereafter, macrolides were shown to exert immunomodulatory effects on a wide range of cells; epithelial cells, macrophages, monocytes, eosinophils, neutrophils, and lymphocytes. The 14- and 15-membered macrolides are known to lead to suppression of neutrophil chemotaxis and oxidative burst, and inhibition of the release of proinflammatory cytokines from monocytes (Sato et al. 1998, Khan et al. 1999, Rubin and Tamaoki 2000). From the point of view of their unique pharmacological actions, recently we revealed that these macrolides inhibited alpha-toxin-induced events in vivo and in vitro. In this review, we show the mechanism for the action of macrolides on the biological activities of the toxin.

2. Characterization of alpha-toxin

The genes encoding alpha-toxin (Titball et al. 1989), *Bacillus cereus* PLC (BC-PLC) (Gilmore et al. 1989), and PLCs from *C. bifermentans* (Tso and Siebel 1989) and *Listeria monocytogenes* (Vazquez-Boland et al. 1992) have been isolated and their nucleotide sequences were determined. (Titball 1993). It therefore was found that the deduced amino acid sequences of alpha-toxin and these enzymes exhibit significant homology up to approximately 250 residues from the N-terminus. Therefore, the findings show that alpha-toxin (370 amino acid residues) belongs to the PLC family. BC-PLC has two tightly bound and one loosely bound zinc ions (Hough et al. 1989, Vallee and Auld 1993). Crystallographic and site-directed mutagenesis analysis of alpha-toxin revealed that one zinc ion is tightly coordinated with His-11 and Asp-130, a second is coordinated tightly with His-148 and loosely with Glu-152, and a divalent cation is loosely associated with His-68, -126, -136 and Asp-130 (Nagahama et al. 1995, Nagahama et al. 1996b) and that Asp-56 is essential for catalytic activity (Nagahama et al. 1997), indicating that the catalytic site of the toxin is located in the N-terminal domain. Furthermore, the crystallographic study indicated that the structure is divided into two domains (Naylor et al. 1998): the N-domain (250 residues), consisting of nine tightly packed α-helices, and the C-domain (120 residues), consisting of an eight-stranded anti-parallel β-sandwich motif. It was confirmed that the N-domain has a structural topology similar to the entire BC-PLC (Hough et al. 1989) and three divalent cations containing zinc ions in the active site, and that amino acid residues involved in zinc-coordination are essential for the enzymatic activities. We reported that mixing the individual N-domain and C-domain restored the hemolytic activity (Nagahama et al. 2002), suggesting that the C-domain affects the activity of the N-domain. Guillouard *et al.* (Guillouard et al. 1997) and Naylor *et al.* (Naylor et al. 1998) reported that the fold of the C-domain is similar to those of the "C2" and "C2-like" domains, present in eukaryotic proteins involved in signal transduction, of eukaryotic phospholipid-binding proteins such as synaptotagmin. Guillouard *et al.* (Guillouard et al. 1997) reported that the C-domain of alpha-toxin mediates interactions with membrane phospholipids in a calcium-dependent manner. Furthermore, Alape-Giron *et al.* (Alape-Giron et al. 2000) reported that Tyr-275, -307 and -331 residues are critical for binding of the toxin. We also reported that acrylodan-labeled C-domain variants (S263C and S365C) bound to liposomes and internalized into the hydrophobic environment in liposomes (Nagahama et al. 2002, Nagahama, Michiue and Sakurai 1996a). It therefore appears that the C-domain plays an important role in binding to membranes. From these observations, it is apparent that alpha-toxin consists of two distinct modules: the N-domain catalyses phospholipid hydrolysis in membranes and the C-domain binds to and inserts into membranes (Fig. 1)

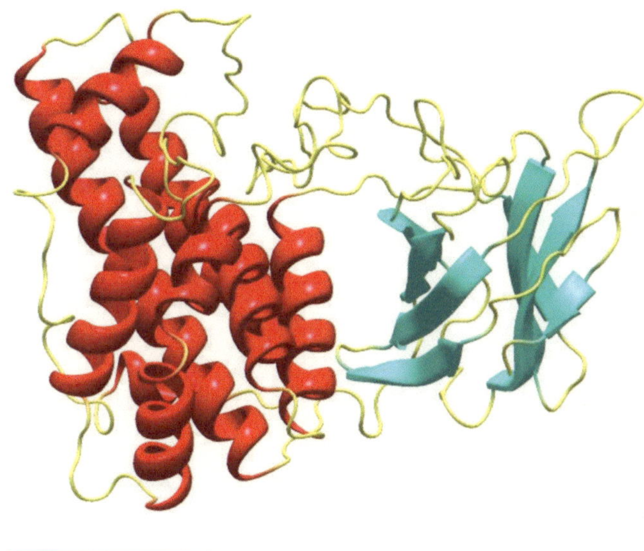

Fig. 1. Structure of *Clostridium perfringens* alpha-toxin

3. The action of *Clostridium perfringens* alpha-toxin

3.1 The effect of pro-inflammatory cytokines on alpha-toxin-induced death

Cytokines are small proteins involved in key events of the inflammatory process. Beutler et al. reported that neutralization of TNF- α released by the intravenous injection of a lethal dose of lipopolysaccharide (LPS) prevented death in mice (Beutler, Milsark and Cerami 1985). Later, Tracey et al. demonstrated that a monoclonal anti-TNF- α antibody protected baboons against sepsis elicited by *Escherichia coli* (Tracey et al. 1987). It has been reported that the overproduction of inflammatory cytokines induced by shiga toxin (van Setten et al. 1996, Yoshimura et al. 1997) and LPS (Palsson-McDermott and O'Neill 2004) led to a cytokine storm, damaging various cells and tissues. Stevens et al. and Bunting et al. suggested that alpha-toxin contributed to shock by stimulating production of endogenous mediators such as TNF- α and platelet-activating factor (Bunting et al. 1997, Stevens and Bryant 1997). Fig. 2 shows that intravenous injection of alpha-toxin in mice resulted in the release of TNF- α, interleukin (IL)-1β, IL-6, IL-10, IFN-γ, and IL-2 in serum (Fig. 2), and eventually death. TNF- α, IL-1β, and IL-6 are known to be important elements in the inflammatory response. Therefore, it is possible that the lethality of alpha-toxin is associated with the release of these inflammatory cytokines.

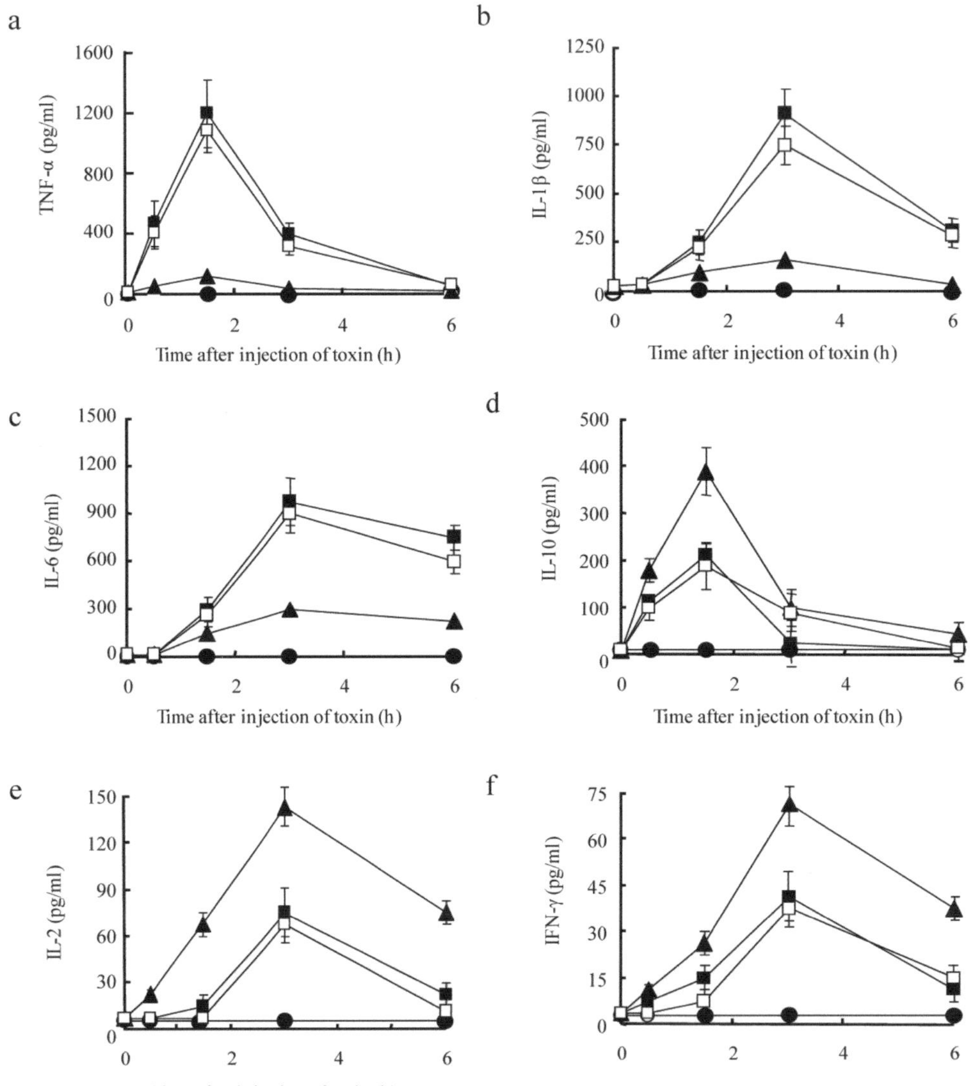

Fig. 2. Effect of macrolide antibiotics on the toxin-induced release of cytokines in blood of mice Mice received ERM or KTM for 5 days every 24 h and were injected intravenously with 20 ng of alpha-toxin. Cytokines (TNF-α, IL-1β, IL-6, IL-10, IFN-γ and IL-2) in the blood were assayed with ELISA kits. Symbols: control, •; Saline + alpha-toxin, ■; ERM (0.5 mg/mouse) + alpha-toxin; ▲; KTM (0.5 mg/mouse) + alpha-toxin, □.

To examine the role of inflammatory cytokines in the death caused by the toxin, mice were intravenously injected with the toxin after the administration of an anti-TNF-α, IL-1β, or IL-6 antibody. Untreated mice began to die within 10 hr after the administration of the toxin and all mice died within 12 hr. The survival rate of anti-TNF-α antibody-preinjected mice was 100 and 80% after 8 and 12 hr, respectively, under the conditions (Fig. 3). The anti-IL-1β and anti-IL-6 antibodies had little effect on the lethality (Fig. 3). From the result, it is likely that the lethality of the toxin is related to the release of TNF-α, not of IL-1β or IL-6. To confirm this, the effect of the toxin on TNF-α-deficient mice was tested (Fig. 4). The administration of alpha-toxin killed all of the wild-type mice within 12 h. The survival rate of the TNF-α-knockout mice was 100% and 75% within 12 and 24 h, respectively, consistent with the result obtained by injection of the anti-TNF-α antibody in mice. The observations showed that TNF-α released by the toxin is important in the death caused by the toxin. On the other hand, TNF-α in the range of concentrations found in mice treated with alpha-toxin was not lethal. Therefore, it is apparent that TNF-α alone did not participate in the death from alpha-toxin under our experimental condition. It is likely that TNF-α released by alpha-toxin plays a role in enhancing the actions of the toxin in vivo, but is not a major factor. Therefore, we cannot exclude the possibility that a TNF-α inhibitor is worth pursuing as a novel therapeutic approach to the treatment of gas gangrene and septicemia caused by the microorganism.

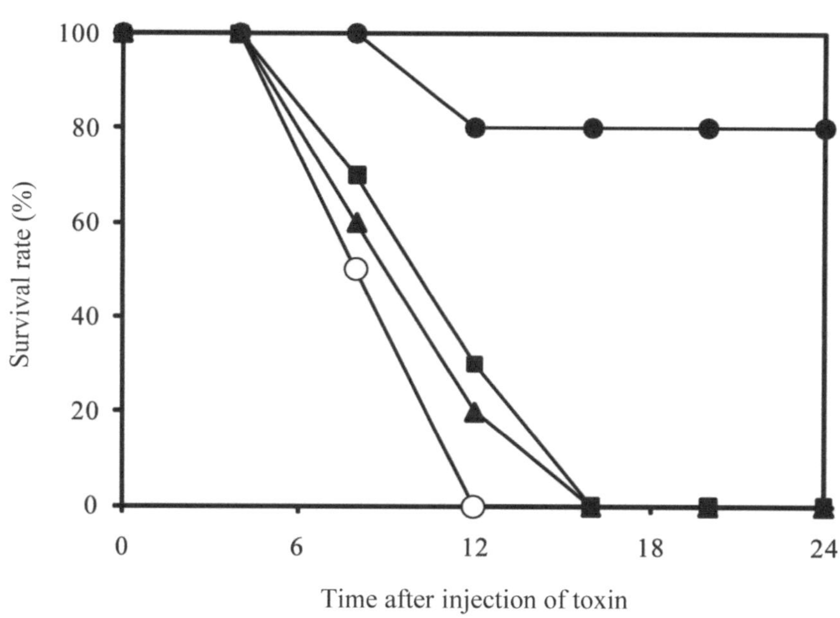

Fig. 3 Effect of anti-TNF-α -IL-1β and -IL-6 antibodies on the lethality of alpha-toxin. Mice received 50 μg of anti-TNF-α, anti-IL-1β, or anti-IL-6 antibody, and after 2 h, were injected intravenously with 20 ng of alpha-toxin. Survival of the mice was monitored at the indicated times after the injection of the toxin. Symbols: Saline + alpha-toxin, ○; anti-TNF-α antibody + alpha-toxin, •; anti-IL-1β antibody + alpha-toxin, ▲; anti-IL-6 antibody + alpha-toxin, ■.

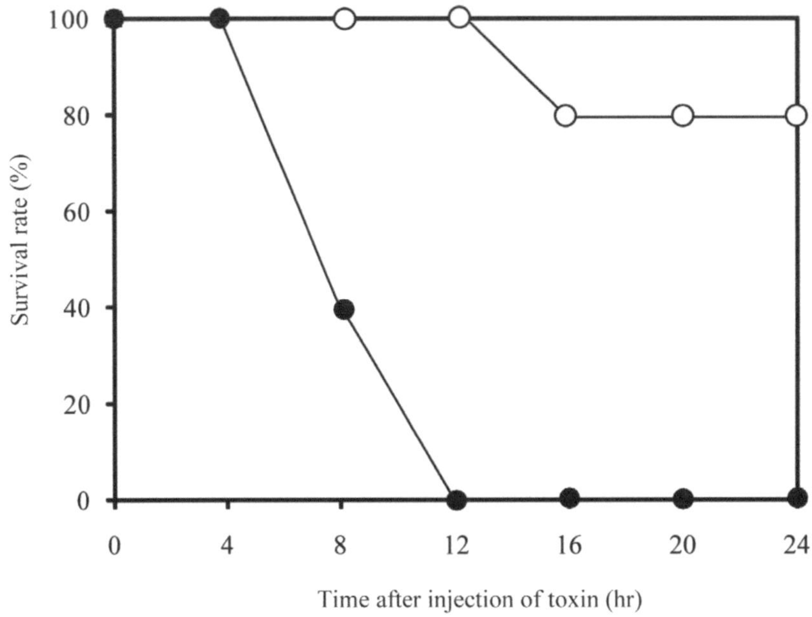

Fig. 4. Comparision of the lethality of alpha-toxin in wild-type mice and TNF-α knockout mice Mice were injected intravenously with 20 ng of alpha-toxin. Survival of the mice was monitored at the indicated times after the injection. Symbols: control mouse (B10D2), •; TNF-α knockout mouse, ○.

4. The potency of macrolide antibiotics

4.1 The effect on alpha-toxin-induced death

Macrolides, particularly those derived from 14- and 15-membered rings, exert anti-infammatory effects through a variety of signaling pathways including activator protein-1 (AP-1) and nuclear factor-kappaB (NF-κB) (Sato et al. 1998, Khan et al. 1999, Desaki et al. 2000, Rubin and Tamaoki 2000, Kikuchi et al. 2002). The antibiotics have been reported to impair the production of pro-inflammatory cytokines (Kadota et al. 1993, Fujii et al. 1995). Abe et al. reported that macrolides repressed IL-8 gene expression by suppressing both AP-1 binding sites and NF-κB (Abe et al. 2000). Shchultz et al. postulated that the treatment with macrolides results in suppression of the production of TNF-α and granulocyte-macrophage colony-stimulating factor (Schultz et al. 1998). Simpson et al. have also reported that 14- and 15-member macrolide antibiotics attenuated the activation of neutrophils induced by various inflammatory stimuli (Simpson et al. 2008).

We measured the release of these cytokines induced by the toxin in mice preinjected with the 14-membered macrolide, ERM or the 16-membered, KTM. In mice preinjected with ERM, the toxin-induced release of pro-inflammatory cytokines, TNF- α, IL-1β, and IL-6, in blood was markedly decreased (Fig. 2), whereas the toxin-induced release of the T-helper type 1 (Th1) cytokines, IFN-γ and IL-2, and the T-helper type 2 (Th2) cytokine, IL-10, increased approximately 2-fold, compared with that in mice preinjected with ERM (Fig. 2). The action of AZM resembled that of ERM. In mice preinjected with KTM, the toxin-induced release of these cytokines was the same as that in the control mice. The administration of

ERM or KTM alone caused no release of these cytokines. It therefore is apparent that ERM and AZM inhibit the toxin-induced release of pro-inflammatory cytokines, and enhance that of Th1 and Th2 cytokines in vivo. It is interesting that the antibiotics increased levels of Th1 and Th2 cytokines under the conditions. The antibiotics may control a balance of the immune system disrupted by the toxin.

We examined the effect of ERM, AZM, and KTM on the toxin-induced death. Alpha-toxin-injected mice began to die after about 8 hr, and all mice died within 12 hr of the administration (Fig. 5). ERM- or AZM-preinjected mice survived up to 18 hr after the injection of alpha-toxin. The survival rate of mice preinjected with ERM and AZM was about 80 and 70%, respectively, 24 h after the administration of the toxin, showing that ERM and AZM inhibited the toxin's lethal effect. These results show that the 14-ring and the 15-ring macrolides have inhibitory effects on the lethality of alpha-toxin, but the 16-ring macrolides do not. The result coincided with that reported previously (Oda et al. 2008).

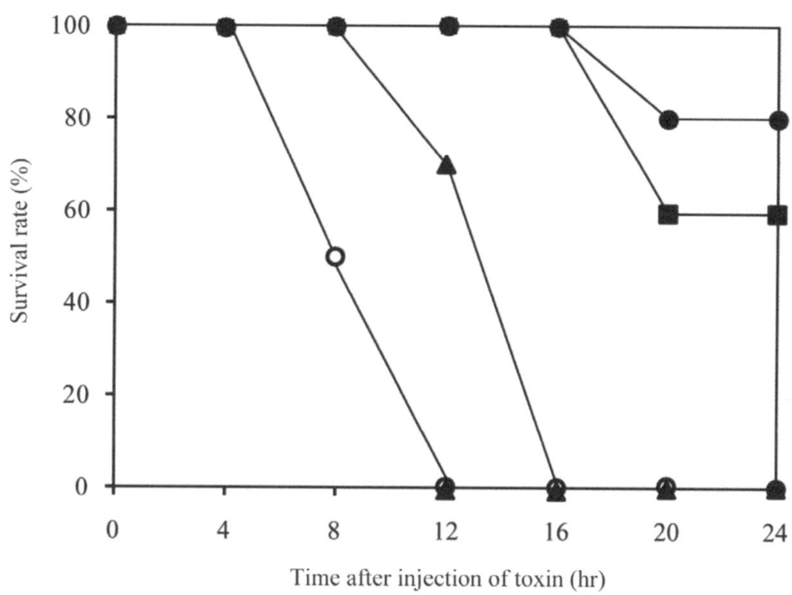

Fig. 5. Effect of macrolide antibiotics on the lethality of alpha-toxin
Mice received 15 mg/kg of ERM, AZM, or KTM for 5 days every 24 h, and were then injected intravenously with 20 ng of alpha-toxin. Survival of the mice was monitored every 4 hr after the injection of the toxin. Symbols: Saline + alpha-toxin, ○; ERM + alpha-toxin, •; AZM + alpha-toxin, ■; KTM + alpha-toxin, ▲.

4.2 Effect on systemic hemolysis induced by alpha-toxin

Massive intravascular hemolysis is reported to be diagnostic of *C. perfringens* septicemia (Alvarez et al. 1999). Bunderen et al. reported that the disease occurs in immunocompromised patients and patients with underlying malignancy, or in otherwise healthy individuals with abdominal surgery or following abortion (van Bunderen et al. 2010). Combination therapy with penicillin and clindamycin has been shown to minimally improve survival in animal studies (Stevens et al. 1987). However, at present, the treatment of choice for *C. perfringens* septicemia is intravenously administered high-dose penicillin and surgical debridement of infectious focus. It is reported that early treatment can rescue patients from an otherwise rapidly fatal outcome, and that the disease with massive hemolysis leads to death within a few hours (Alvarez et al. 1999). Bunderen et al. also found that the toxin-induced hemolysis is an additional prominent factor in the pathogenesis of septicemia caused by *C. perfringens* (van Bunderen et al. 2010).

We have reported the relationship between the toxin-induced hemolysis and activation of phospholipid metabolism via pertussis toxin-sensitive GTP-binding protein (Gi) (Sakurai, Ochi and Tanaka 1994, Ochi et al. 1996, Ochi et al. 2004, Oda et al. 2008). Intravenous injection of alpha-toxin in mice resulted in massive intravascular hemolysis (Sugahara and Osaka 1970, Kreidl, Green and Wren 2002). However, little is known about the mechanism of hemolysis induced by the toxin in vivo. We investigated the effect of cytokines on the hemolysis induced by alpha-toxin. Mouse erythrocytes were treated with a sub-hemolytic dose of alpha-toxin at 37°C for 30 min, and then incubated with various concentrations of TNF-α, IL-1β or IL-6 for 60 min. Fig. 6 shows that TNF-α enhanced the toxin-induced hemolysis of mouse erythrocytes in a dose-dependent manner, but IL-1β and IL-6 did not.

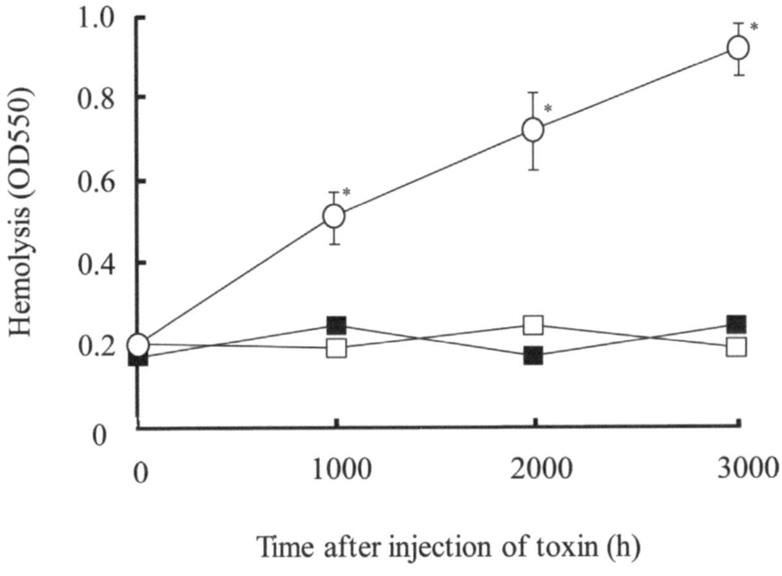

Fig. 6. Effect of cytokines on hemolysis induced by alpha-toxin in mouse erythrocytes
The washed erythrocytes of mice were incubated with 20 ng/mL of alpha-toxin at 37°C for 30 min, and then treated with various concentrations of cytokines at 37°C for 60 min. Symbols: TNF-α, ○; IL-1β, □; IL-6; ■. *, $p < 0.01$.

To investigate the effect of ERM and KTM on the hemolysis induced by alpha-toxin in vivo, mice preinjected with ERM and KTM were intravenously administered the toxin. The alpha-toxin-induced hemolysis was markedly decreased in the ERM- or AZM-injected mice, but not KTM-injected mice (Fig. 7). Blockage of TNF-α's release by ERM or AZM in vivo paralleled the reduction in hemolysis caused by the toxin. It therefore appears that TNF-α enhances the toxin-induced hemolysis in vivo, suggesting that ERM and AZM are effective against the systemic hemolysis induced by alpha-toxin. The result suggests that the antibiotics may prevent hemolytic anemia induced by the toxin.

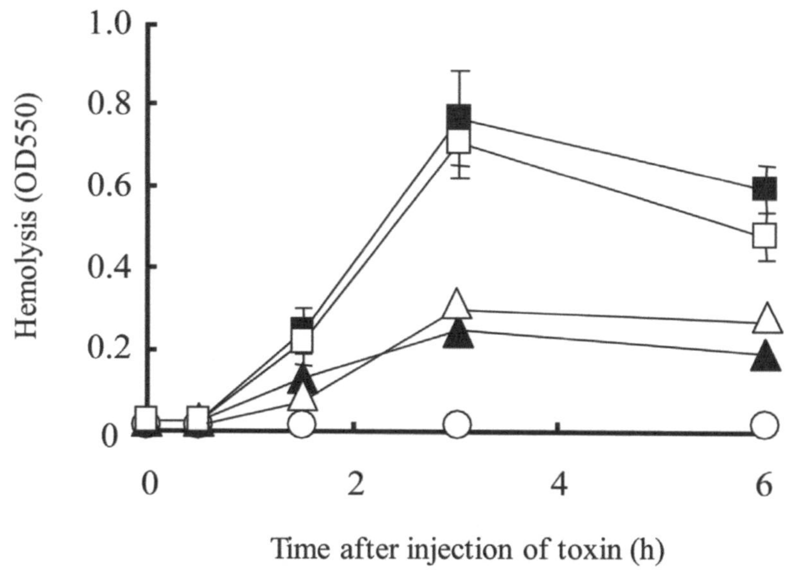

Fig. 7. Hemolysis induced by alpha-toxin in mice pretreated with macrolide antibiotics Mice received various concentrations of ERM or KTM for 5 days every 24 h, and were then injected intravenously with 20 ng of alpha-toxin. The amount of hemoglobin in the blood was measured spectrophotometrically. Symbols: control, ○; Saline + alpha-toxin, □; ERM (0.5 mg/mouse) + alpha-toxin; ▲; AZM (0.5 mg/mouse) + alpha-toxin; Δ, KTM (0.5 mg/mouse) + alpha-toxin, ■.

4.3 The effect on alpha-toxin-induced activation of neutrophils

Alpha-toxin induced the release of TNF-α from neutrophils and macrophages. The 14- and 15-membered macrolides inhibited the toxin-induced release of TNF-α, IL-1β, and IL-6 in vivo, as mentioned above. Furthermore, the macrolides prevented the toxin-induced activation of phagocytes and release of TNF-α from cells in vitro. We investigated the effect of the toxin on neutrophils isolated from the macrolide-preinjected mice. The release of TNF-α induced by the toxin from neutrophils prepared from ERM- or AZM-preinjected mice was about 20% of that from neutrophils of untreated mice (Fig. 8A). Little significant reduction in the amount of TNF-α released was observed in neutrophils from mice pretreated with KTM, compared with the control (Fig. 8A). Furthermore, the pretreatment of macrophages with ERM and AZM in vivo resulted in a reduction in the toxin-induced release of TNF-α, but that with KTM did not. It therefore appears that the treatment of these phagocytes with ERM and AZM resulted in a reduction in the response to the toxin.

We have reported the mechanism for activation of neutrophils by the toxin as follows (Fig. 8B). Alpha-toxin stimulated the generation of O_2^- in rabbit neutrophils in vitro (Ochi et al. 2002, Oda et al. 2006). Treatment of neutrophils with the toxin resulted in tyrosine phosphorylation of a protein of about 140 kDa (Fig. 8C). The protein reacted with an anti-tyrosine kinase A (TrkA) antibody and bound nerve growth factor (NGF). The anti-TrkA antibody inhibited the toxin-induced production of O_2^- from the cells and binding of the toxin to the protein. In addition, the toxin did not bind to PC12 cells treated with TrkA-siRNA, which did not express TrkA. The observations show that the TrkA is a receptor of alpha-toxin. The toxin induced phosphorylation of 3-phosphoinositide-dependent protein kinase 1 (PDK1), which functions as a downstream mediator of TrkA. K252a, an inhibitor of TrkA, and LY294002, an inhibitor of phosphatidylinositol 3-kinase (PI3K), reduced the toxin-induced production of O_2^- and phosphorylation of PDK1, but not the formation of diacylglycerol (DG) (Fig. 8D). These inhibitors inhibited the toxin-induced phosphorylation

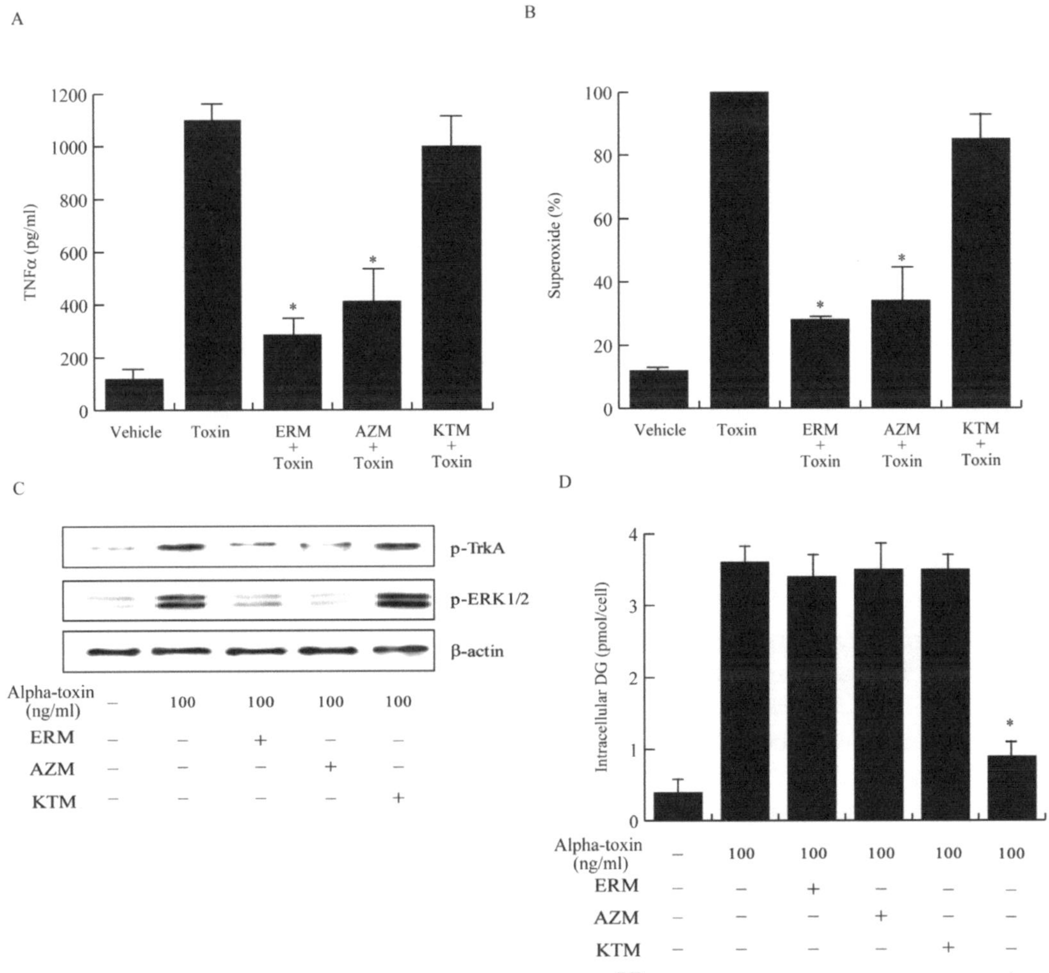

Fig. 8. Effect of alpha-toxin on TrkA-mediated signal transduction in neutrophils prepared from mice preinjected with macrolides

Neutrophils were prepared from mice injected with ERM, AZM, or KTM. A) The neutrophils were incubated with 100 ng of alpha-toxin at 37°C for 3 h. The release of TNF-α was assayed with an ELISA kit. *, $p < 0.01$. B) Production of O_2^- was monitored for 15 min based on MCLA-chemiluminescence. O_2^- production induced by alpha-toxin alone was set as the maximal response (100%). *, $p < 0.05$. C) The neutrophils were incubated with 100 ng/ml of alpha-toxin at 37°C for 10 min, and subjected to SDS-PAGE and Western blotting using specific antibody. D) The neutrophils were incubated with 100 ng/ml of alpha-toxin at 37°C for 10 min, and DG in the cells was measured. *, $p < 0.01$.

of protein kinase C θ (PKCθ). On the other hand, U73122, a PLC inhibitor, and pertussis toxin inhibited the toxin-induced generation of O_2^- and formation of DG, but not the phosphorylation of TrkA and PDK1 (Fig. 8D). These observations show that the toxin independently induces production of DG through activation of endogenous phosphatidylinositol PI-PLC via Gi and phosphorylation of PDK1 via the TrkA signaling pathway and the two events synergistically activate PKCθ which is involved in the generation of O_2^- through the stimulation of mitogen-activated protein kinase (MAPK)-associated signaling events (Fig. 9).

Macrolide antibiotics have been reported to inhibit effects through signaling pathways including NF-κB and AP-1. It has been reported that ERM, clarithromycin, and

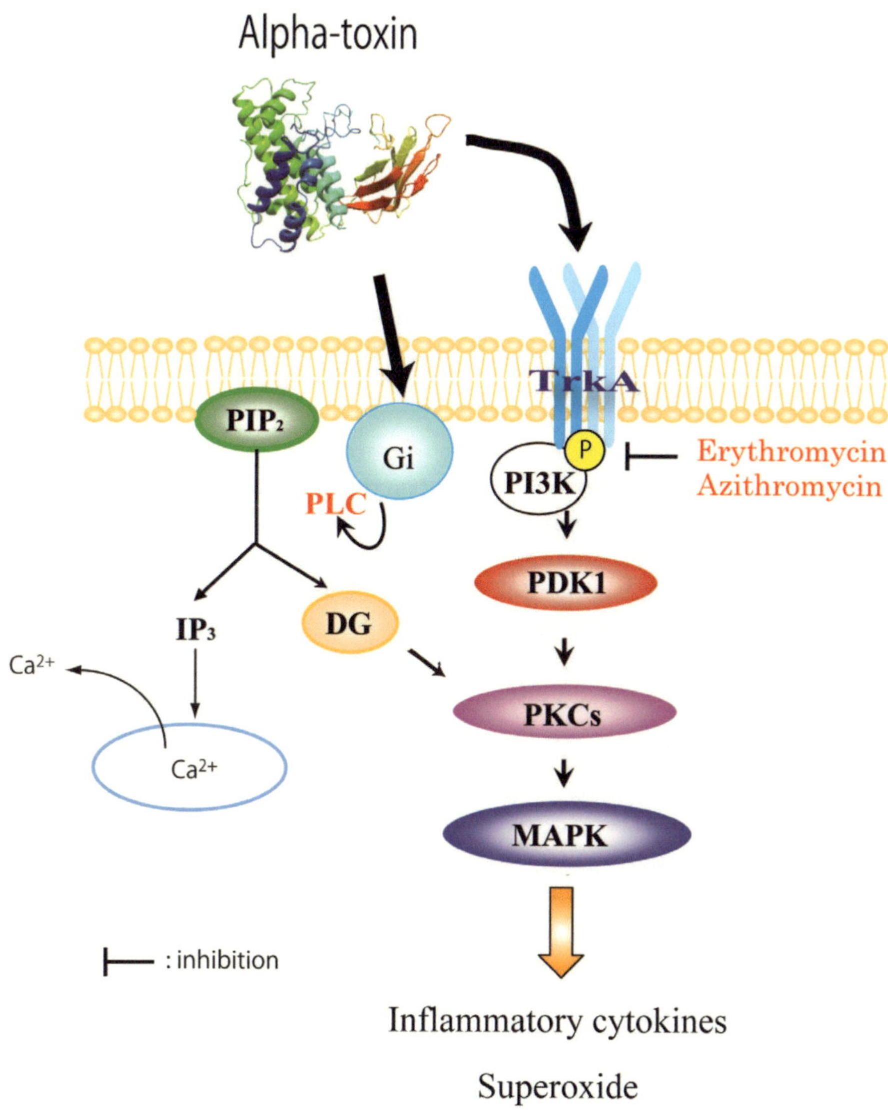

Fig. 9. Effect of ERM and AZM on alpha-toxin-activated signal transduction

roxithromycin inhibit the generation of O_2^- by stimulus-activated neutrophils (Anderson 1989, Hand and King-Thompson 1990). However, little is known about the inhibitory mechanism of the antibiotics. Recently we revealed that macrolides prevent the toxin-induced death, production of O_2^-, and release of TNF-α in neutrophils through inactivation of TrkA (Oda et al. 2008). ERM and AZM inhibited the toxin-induced phosphorylation of TrkA under conditions in which the toxin inhibits biological activities; production of O_2^- and release of TNF-α (Fig. 8). On the other hand, treatment with ERM and AZM had no effect on the formation of DG via Gi in rabbit neutrophils treated with alpha-toxin. KTM, which does not inhibit the biological activities of the toxin, did not prevent them. These observations provided evidence that inhibition of the toxin-induced phosphorylation of TrkA by ERM and AZM results in suppression of activation of neutrophils, formation of O_2^-, and release of TNF-α. Therefore, the results show that 14- and 15-membered macrolides specifically inhibit the phosphorylation of TrkA, viz. activation of the protein.

5. Discussion

C. perfringens alpha-toxin causes death, hemolysis, the activation of neutrophils, and the release of TNF-α through activation of MAPK-associated signaling via two pathways, activation of endogenous PI-PLC via Gi and PDK1 via phsophorylation of TrkA. The 14- and 15-membered macrolides specifically inhibited the phosphorylation of TrkA, preventing the activation of the MAPK signaling pathway present in the downstream region of TrkA. Therefore, it was found that the antibiotics specifically block these activities of the toxin by inhibiting the phosphorylation of TrkA.

TNF-α appears to play an important role in the lethal effect of the toxin, because 1) the anti-TNF-α antibody prevented death caused by the toxin, 2) TNF-α-knockout mice were resistant to the toxin, and 3) the 14- and 15-membered macrolides, which prevent the release of TNF-α induced by the toxin, inhibited the lethal and hemolytic effects of the toxin. However, Wiersnga and Poll reported that trials with an anti-TNF-α antibody and recombinant IL-1 receptor antagonist for clinical septicemia failed, and many other anti-inflammatory strategies were not successful in altering the outcome of patients with septicemia (Anas et al. 2010). Furthermore, the fallacy of the notion that excessive inflammation is the main or sole underlying cause of an adverse outcome in septic patients has been pointed out in the review by Wiersnga and Poll (Wiersinga and van der Poll 2007). On the other hand, considering that bacteria grow in patients with septicemia, there are many unanswered questions about the immune functions of the host, clearance of bacteria in vivo by antimicrobial agents, and surgical resection of foci and so on. Therefore, our findings on the role of TFN-α in diseases caused by *C. perfringens* should be considered significant. Certainly, TNF-α alone in the range of concentrations found in mice treated with alpha-toxin was not lethal. Thus, our results seem that TNF-α promotes lethality and massive intravascular hemolysis caused by the toxin. Fourteen- and the 15-membered macrolides have been shown to exert immunomodulatory effects on a wide range of cells; epithelial cells, macrophages, monocytes, eosinophils, neutrophils, and lymphocytes. The antibiotics are known to inhibit adherence, oxidative burst, cytokine expression and mobility. The administration of the 14- and 15-membered macrolides resulted in a drastic reduction in alpha-toxin-induced release of proinflammatory cytokines and systemic hemolysis and death, and increases in Th 1 and 2 cytokines in mice treated with the toxin. Yan et al. reported that lysophosphatidylcholine (LPC) induced a modest and transient change in the levels of certain cytokines and that the Th 1 cytokines, IFN-γ, IL-2 and IL-12, were increased in response to LPC, whereas the proinflammatory cytokines, TNF-α and IL-1β, were decreased (Yan et al. 2004), showing that the pattern of cytokine regulation induced by alpha-toxin in mice treated with the macrolides is similar to that observed in the LPC-treated LPS model. Increases in Th 1 cytokines, as well as the combined decrease of TNF-α and IL-1β, have been reported to have beneficial effects in sepsis (Weighardt et al. 2002, Nakahata et al. 2001). Yan et al. did not exclude the possibility that the combined effect of all these changes in cytokines may contribute to improved survival (Yan et al. 2004). Our result concerning the behavior of proinflammatory cytokines was consistent with that reported by others. On the basis of these findings, a careful balance between the inflammatory and anti-inflammatory response appears to be significant for survival in patients with septicemia. Therefore, it is possible that macrolides are valuable in patients with septicemia caused by *C. perfringens*.

The 14- and 15- member-macrolide antibiotics are effective in the treatment of infectious diseases caused by *C. perfringens*, but not in excluding *C. perfringens* from foci under the conditions. Highly effective antimicrobial agents against *C. perfringens* are required for treatment of the diseases.

6. Conclusion

C. perfringens alpha-toxin, the main agent involved in the development of gas gangrene and septicemia, induces death, hemolysis, necrosis and the activation of macrophages and neutrophils. The toxin elicits these activities through the activation of an intracellular signaling pathway involving MAPK-associated signal transduction from Gi and/or TrkA. The 14- and 15-membered macrolides specifically blocked the phosphorylaion of TrkA, inhibiting these toxin-induced activities. It therefore appears that the macrolide antibiotics are effective in an improvement in clinical symptoms caused by *C. perfringens*. However, growth rates of *C. perfringens* are known to be significantly higher in infectious foci without neutrophils. The macrolides are likely not to be effective in inhibiting the growth of *C. perfringens* under the conditions. Penicillins are known to be highly effective in preventing the growth of microorganisms. In conclusion, treatment with 14- and 15-membered macrolides, an inhibitor of alpha-toxin, and high doses of penicillins, antimicrobial agents, would be effective against diseases caused by *C. perfringens*.

7. References

Abe, S., H. Nakamura, S. Inoue, H. Takeda, H. Saito, S. Kato, N. Mukaida, K. Matsushima & H. Tomoike (2000) Interleukin-8 gene repression by clarithromycin is mediated by the activator protein-1 binding site in human bronchial epithelial cells. *Am J Respir Cell Mol Biol*, 22, 51-60. ISSN pp. 1044-1549

Alape-Giron, A., M. Flores-Diaz, I. Guillouard, C. E. Naylor, R. W. Titball, A. Rucavado, B. Lomonte, A. K. Basak, J. M. Gutierrez, S. T. Cole & M. Thelestam (2000) Identification of residues critical for toxicity in *Clostridium perfringens* phospholipase C, the key toxin in gas gangrene. *Eur J Biochem,* 267, pp. 5191-5197. ISSN 0014-2956

Aldridge, A. J. (2002) Role of the neutrophil in septic shock and the adult respiratory distress syndrome. *Eur J Surg,* 168, pp. 204-214.

Alvarez, A., S. Rives, B. Nomdedeu & A. Pereira (1999) Massive hemolysis in *Clostridium perfringens* infection. *Haematologica,* 84, pp. 571-573. ISSN 0390-6078

Anas, A. A., W. J. Wiersinga, A. F. de Vos & T. van der Poll (2010) Recent insights into the pathogenesis of bacterial sepsis. *Neth J Med,* 68, pp. 147-152. ISSN 1872-9061

Anderson, R. (1989) Erythromycin and roxithromycin potentiate human neutrophil locomotion in vitro by inhibition of leukoattractant-activated superoxide generation and autooxidation. *J Infect Dis,* 159, pp. 966-973.

Awad, M. M., D. M. Ellemor, R. L. Boyd, J. J. Emmins & J. I. Rood (2001) Synergistic effects of alpha-toxin and perfringolysin O in *Clostridium perfringens*-mediated gas gangrene. *Infect Immun,* 69, pp. 7904-7910. ISSN 0019-9567

Beutler, B., I. W. Milsark & A. C. Cerami (1985) Passive immunization against cachectin/tumor necrosis factor protects mice from lethal effect of endotoxin. *Science,* 229, pp. 869-871. ISSN 0036-8075

Bryant, A. E., R. Y. Chen, Y. Nagata, Y. Wang, C. H. Lee, S. Finegold, P. H. Guth & D. L. Stevens (2000) Clostridial gas gangrene. I. Cellular and molecular mechanisms of microvascular dysfunction induced by exotoxins of *Clostridium perfringens. J Infect Dis,* 182, pp. 799-807.

Bryant, A. E. & D. L. Stevens (1996) Phospholipase C and perfringolysin O from *Clostridium perfringens* upregulate endothelial cell-leukocyte adherence molecule 1 and intercellular leukocyte adherence molecule 1 expression and induce interleukin-8 synthesis in cultured human umbilical vein endothelial cells. *Infect Immun,* 64, pp. 358-362.

Bunting, M., D. E. Lorant, A. E. Bryant, G. A. Zimmerman, T. M. McIntyre, D. L. Stevens & S. M. Prescott (1997) Alpha toxin from *Clostridium perfringens* induces proinflammatory changes in endothelial cells. *J Clin Invest,* 100, pp. 565-574.

Calandra, T., P. Y. Bochud & D. Heumann (2002) Cytokines in septic shock. *Curr Clin Top Infect Dis,* 22, pp. 1-23.

Desaki M., H. Takizawa, T. Ohtoshi, T. Kasama, K. Kobayashi, T. Sunazuka, S. Omura, K. Yamamoto & K. Ito (2000) Erythromycin suppresses nuclear factor-kB and activator protein-1 activation in human bronchial epithelial cells. *Biochem Biophys Res Commun.* 267, pp. 124-128.

Dinarello, C. A. (2004) Therapeutic strategies to reduce IL-1 activity in treating local and systemic inflammation. *Curr Opin Pharmacol,* 4, pp. 378-385.

Ellemor, D. M., R. N. Baird, M. M. Awad, R. L. Boyd, J. I. Rood & J. J. Emmins (1999) Use of genetically manipulated strains of *Clostridium perfringens* reveals that both alpha-toxin and theta-toxin are required for vascular leukostasis to occur in experimental gas gangrene. *Infect Immun,* 67, pp. 4902-4907. ISSN 0019-9567

Fujii, T., J. Kadota, K. Kawakami, K. Iida, R. Shirai, M. Kaseda, S. Kawamoto & S. Kohno (1995) Long term effect of erythromycin therapy in patients with chronic *Pseudomonas aeruginosa* infection. *Thorax,* 50, pp. 1246-1252.

Gilmore, M. S., A. L. Cruz-Rodz, M. Leimeister-Wachter, J. Kreft & W. Goebel (1989) A Bacillus cereus cytolytic determinant, cereolysin AB, which comprises the phospholipase C and sphingomyelinase genes: nucleotide sequence and genetic linkage. *J Bacteriol*, 171, pp. 744-753. ISSN 0021-9193

Guillouard, I., P. M. Alzari, B. Saliou & S. T. Cole (1997) The carboxy-terminal C2-like domain of the alpha-toxin from *Clostridium perfringens* mediates calcium-dependent membrane recognition. *Mol Microbiol*, 26, pp. 867-876. ISSN 0950-382X

Hand, W. L. & N. L. King-Thompson (1990) Uptake of antibiotics by human polymorphonuclear leukocyte cytoplasts. *Antimicrob Agents Chemother*, 34, pp. 1189-1193. ISSN 0066-4804

Hough, E., L. K. Hansen, B. Birknes, K. Jynge, S. Hansen, A. Hordvik, C. Little, E. Dodson & Z. Derewenda (1989) High-resolution (1.5 A) crystal structure of phospholipase C from *Bacillus cereus*. *Nature*, 338, pp. 357-360. ISSN 0028-0836

Kadota, J., O. Sakito, S. Kohno, H. Sawa, H. Mukae, H. Oda, K. Kawakami, K. Fukushima, K. Hiratani & K. Hara (1993) A mechanism of erythromycin treatment in patients with diffuse panbronchiolitis. *Am Rev Respir Dis*, 147, pp. 153-159.

Khan, A. A., T. R. Slifer, F. G. Araujo & J. S. Remington (1999) Effect of clarithromycin and azithromycin on production of cytokines by human monocytes. *Int J Antimicrob Agents*, 11, pp. 121-132.

Kikuchi T, K. Hagiwara, Y. Honda, K. Gomi, T. Kobayashi, H. Takahashi, Y. Tokue, A. Watanabe & T. Nukiwa. (2002) Clarithromycin suppresses lipopolysaccharide-induced interleukin-8 production by human monocytes through AP-1 and NF-κB transcription factors. *J Antimicrob Chemother*, 49, pp.745–55.

Kreidl, K. O., G. R. Green & S. M. Wren (2002) Intravascular hemolysis from a *Clostridium perfringens* liver abscess. *J Am Coll Surg*, 194, pp. 387. ISSN 1072-7515

Lum, L., B. R. Wong, R. Josien, J. D. Becherer, H. Erdjument-Bromage, J. Schlondorff, P. Tempst, Y. Choi & C. P. Blobel (1999) Evidence for a role of a tumor necrosis factor-alpha (TNF-alpha)-converting enzyme-like protease in shedding of TRANCE, a TNF family member involved in osteoclastogenesis and dendritic cell survival. *J Biol Chem*, 274, pp. 13613-13618.

Nagahama, M., K. Michiue & J. Sakurai (1996a) Membrane-damaging action of *Clostridium perfringens* alpha-toxin on phospholipid liposomes. *Biochim Biophys Acta*, 1280, pp. 120-126.

Nagahama, M., M. Mukai, S. Morimitsu, S. Ochi & J. Sakurai (2002) Role of the C-domain in the biological activities of *Clostridium perfringens* alpha-toxin. *Microbiol Immunol*, 46, pp. 647-655.

Nagahama, M., T. Nakayama, K. Michiue & J. Sakurai (1997) Site-specific mutagenesis of *Clostridium perfringens* alpha-toxin: replacement of Asp-56, Asp-130, or Glu-152 causes loss of enzymatic and hemolytic activities. *Infect Immun*, 65, pp. 3489-3492.

Nagahama, M., S. Ochi, K. Kobayashi & J. Sakurai (1996b) The relationship between histidine residues and various biological activities of *Clostridium perfringens* alpha toxin. *Adv Exp Med Biol*, 391, pp. 251-255. ISSN 0065-2598

Nagahama, M., Y. Okagawa, T. Nakayama, E. Nishioka & J. Sakurai (1995) Site-directed mutagenesis of histidine residues in *Clostridium perfringens* alpha-toxin. *J Bacteriol,* 177, pp. 1179-1185.

Nakahata, E., Y. Shindoh, T. Takayama & C. Shindoh (2001) Interleukin-12 prevents diaphragm muscle deterioration in a septic animal model. *Comp Biochem Physiol A Mol Integr Physiol,* 130, pp. 653-663. ISSN 1095-6433

Naylor, C. E., J. T. Eaton, A. Howells, N. Justin, D. S. Moss, R. W. Titball & A. K. Basak (1998) Structure of the key toxin in gas gangrene. *Nat Struct Biol,* 5, pp. 738-746. ISSN 1072-8368

Ochi, S., K. Hashimoto, M. Nagahama & J. Sakurai (1996) Phospholipid metabolism induced by *Clostridium perfringens* alpha-toxin elicits a hot-cold type of hemolysis in rabbit erythrocytes. *Infect Immun,* 64, pp. 3930-3933.

Ochi, S., T. Miyawaki, H. Matsuda, M. Oda, M. Nagahama & J. Sakurai (2002) *Clostridium perfringens* alpha-toxin induces rabbit neutrophil adhesion. *Microbiology,* 148, pp. 237-245.

Ochi, S., M. Oda, H. Matsuda, S. Ikari & J. Sakurai (2004) *Clostridium perfringens* alpha-toxin activates the sphingomyelin metabolism system in sheep erythrocytes. *J Biol Chem,* 279, pp. 12181-12189.

Oda, M., S. Ikari, T. Matsuno, Y. Morimune, M. Nagahama & J. Sakurai (2006) Signal transduction mechanism involved in *Clostridium perfringens* alpha-toxin-induced superoxide anion generation in rabbit neutrophils. *Infect Immun,* 74, pp. 2876-2886.

Oda, M., A. Kihara, H. Yoshioka, Y. Saito, N. Watanabe, K. Uoo, M. Higashihara, M. Nagahama, N. Koide, T. Yokochi & J. Sakurai (2008) Effect of erythromycin on biological activities induced by *Clostridium perfringens* alpha-toxin. *J Pharmacol Exp Ther,* 327, pp. 934-940.

Palsson-McDermott, E. M. & L. A. O'Neill (2004) Signal transduction by the lipopolysaccharide receptor, Toll-like receptor-4. *Immunology,* 113, pp. 153-162. ISSN 0019-2805

Riedemann, N. C., R. F. Guo & P. A. Ward (2003) Novel strategies for the treatment of sepsis. *Nat Med,* 9, pp. 517-524.

Rubin, B. K. & J. Tamaoki (2000) Macrolide antibiotics as biological response modifiers. *Curr Opin Investig Drugs,* 1, pp. 169-172.

Sakurai, J., M. Nagahama & M. Oda (2004) *Clostridium perfringens* alpha-toxin: characterization and mode of action. *J Biochem (Tokyo),* 136, pp. 569-574.

Sakurai, J., S. Ochi & H. Tanaka (1994) Regulation of *Clostridium perfringens* alpha-toxin-activated phospholipase C in rabbit erythrocyte membranes. *Infect Immun,* 62, pp. 717-721. ISSN 0019-9567

Sato, K., M. Suga, T. Akaike, S. Fujii, H. Muranaka, T. Doi, H. Maeda & M. Ando (1998) Therapeutic effect of erythromycin on influenza virus-induced lung injury in mice. *Am J Respir Crit Care Med,* 157, pp. 853-857.

Schmid, E. E. (1971) The macrolide group of antibiotics. Mode of action. *Antibiot Chemother,* 17, pp. 52-66.

Schultz, M. J., P. Speelman, S. Zaat, S. J. van Deventer & T. van der Poll (1998) Erythromycin inhibits tumor necrosis factor alpha and interleukin 6 production induced by heat-killed Streptococcus pneumoniae in whole blood. *Antimicrob Agents Chemother,* 42, pp. 1605-1609. ISSN 0066-4804

Simpson, J. L., H. Powell, M. J. Boyle, R. J. Scott & P. G. Gibson (2008) Clarithromycin targets neutrophilic airway inflammation in refractory asthma. *Am J Respir Crit Care Med,* 177, pp. 148-155. ISSN 1535-4970

Stevens, D. L. (2000) The pathogenesis of clostridial myonecrosis. *Int J Med Microbiol,* 290, pp. 497-502.

Stevens, D. L. & A. E. Bryant (1997) Pathogenesis of *Clostridium perfringens* infection: mechanisms and mediators of shock. *Clin Infect Dis,* 25, pp. 160-164.

Sugahara, T. & A. Osaka (1970) Two molecular forms of *Clostridium perfringens* alpha-toxin associated with lethal, hemolytic and enzymatic activities. *Jpn J Med Sci Biol,* 23, pp. 61-66. Stevens, D.L., B.M. Laine, and J.E. Mitten. (1987) Comparison of single and combination antimicrobial agents for prevention of experimental gas gangrene caused by Clostridium perfringens. Antimicrob. Agents Chemother. 31, pp. 312-316.

Titball, R. W. (1993) Bacterial phospholipases C. *Microbiol Rev,* 57, pp. 347-366. ISSN 0146-0749

Titball, R. W., S. E. Hunter, K. L. Martin, B. C. Morris, A. D. Shuttleworth, T. Rubidge, D. W. Anderson & D. C. Kelly (1989) Molecular cloning and nucleotide sequence of the alpha-toxin (phospholipase C) of *Clostridium perfringens. Infect Immun,* 57, pp. 367-376. ISSN 0019-9567

Tracey, K. J., Y. Fong, D. G. Hesse, K. R. Manogue, A. T. Lee, G. C. Kuo, S. F. Lowry & A. Cerami (1987) Anti-cachectin/TNF monoclonal antibodies prevent septic shock during lethal bacteraemia. *Nature,* 330, pp. 662-664.

Tso, J. Y. & C. Siebel (1989) Cloning and expression of the phospholipase C gene from *Clostridium perfringens* and *Clostridium bifermentans. Infect Immun,* 57, pp. 468-476. ISSN 0019-9567

Vallee, B. L. & D. S. Auld (1993) New perspective on zinc biochemistry: cocatalytic sites in multi-zinc enzymes. *Biochemistry,* 32, pp. 6493-6500. ISSN 0006-2960

van Bunderen, C. C., M. K. Bomers, E. Wesdorp, P. Peerbooms & J. Veenstra (2010) *Clostridium perfringens* septicaemia with massive intravascular haemolysis: a case report and review of the literature. *Neth J Med,* 68, pp. 343-346. ISSN 1872-9061

van Setten, P. A., L. A. Monnens, R. G. Verstraten, L. P. van den Heuvel & V. W. van Hinsbergh (1996) Effects of verocytotoxin-1 on nonadherent human monocytes: binding characteristics, protein synthesis, and induction of cytokine release. *Blood,* 88, pp. 174-183.

Vazquez-Boland, J. A., C. Kocks, S. Dramsi, H. Ohayon, C. Geoffroy, J. Mengaud & P. Cossart (1992) Nucleotide sequence of the lecithinase operon of *Listeria monocytogenes* and possible role of lecithinase in cell-to-cell spread. *Infect Immun,* 60, pp. 219-230. ISSN 0019-9567

Weighardt, H., C. D. Heidecke, A. Westerholt, K. Emmanuilidis, S. Maier, M. Veit, K. Gerauer, E. Matevossian, K. Ulm, J. R. Siewert & B. Holzmann (2002) Impaired monocyte IL-12 production before surgery as a predictive factor for the lethal outcome of postoperative sepsis. *Ann Surg,* 235, pp. 560-567. ISSN 0003-4932

Wiersinga, W. J. & T. van der Poll (2007) Is the septic response good or bad? *Curr Infect Dis Rep,* 9, pp. 366-373. ISSN 1523-3847

Yan, J. J., J. S. Jung, J. E. Lee, J. Lee, S. O. Huh, H. S. Kim, K. C. Jung, J. Y. Cho, J. S. Nam, H. W. Suh, Y. H. Kim & D. K. Song (2004) Therapeutic effects of lysophosphatidylcholine in experimental sepsis. *Nat Med,* 10, pp. 161-167. ISSN 1078-8956

Yoshimura, A., Y. Hara, T. Kaneko & I. Kato (1997) Secretion of IL-1 beta, TNF-alpha, IL-8 and IL-1ra by human polymorphonuclear leukocytes in response to lipopolysaccharides from periodontopathic bacteria. *J Periodontal Res,* 32, pp. 279-286.

13

Hyperbaric Oxygen Therapy in the Treatment of Necrosis and Gangrene

Alexander A. Vitin
University of Washington, Seattle, WA, USA

1. Introduction

Historically, hyperbaric oxygen therapy has been used for treatment of decompression sickness in deep-sea divers. Today, hyperbaric oxygen is commonly used for the treatment of wide variety of surgical and non-surgical conditions, and has persuasively proved its high clinical efficiency in many areas. Currently, established indications include different bacterial (mostly anaerobic) and fungal infections, arterial gas embolism, poorly healing diabetic wounds , osteomyelitis, radiation tissue injury, carbon monoxide poisoning, crush injuries, gangrene, brain abscesses, burns, skin grafts or skin flaps at risk of compromised tissue perfusion, severe anemia, and also conditions like long-standing neurologic deficit, cerebral palsy or autism, and many more. The existing trend of ever-expansion indications to previously untouched areas holds for decades.

The purpose of this review is to examine advantages and disadvantages of the hyperbaric oxygen therapy, and also to explore the underlying physiological mechanisms of the hyperbaric oxygen actions in the ischemic, necrotic and otherwise compromised tissues.

This review will mostly be focused on the discussion of clinical efficacy and practical approach to HBOT use in the treatment of different types of gangrene and necrotizing fasciitis. Role and place of hyperbaric oxygen therapy in the treatment of ischemic and diabetic chronic wounds and ulcers will also be explored.

With currently recommended clinically tested protocols and using contemporary equipment, administration of hyperbaric oxygen therapy is generally considered very safe. However, it is not absolutely innocuous, and certain contraindications, ranged from medical problems to physical abnormalities, while mostly relative, should be carefully considered in every case.

The only absolute contraindication for hyperbaric oxygen therapy is untreated tension pneumothorax. Other contraindications include:

1. Severe chronic obstructive pulmonary disease with carbon dioxide
2. retention, pulmonary blebs, and/or dyspnea with slight exertion; restrictive airway disease (possibility of air trapping with barotraumas ensued)
3. Optic neuritis
4. Acute viral infection
5. Congenital spherocytosis
6. Uncontrolled, acute seizures disorders
7. Upper respiratory tract infection
8. Uncontrolled high fever

9. Pregnancy (questionable)
10. Psychiatric problems
11. History of prior thoracic or ear surgery, which would make it impossible to equalize middle ear pressure or pulmonary pressure (Foster,1992)
12. Concomitant chemotherapy with cis-platinum and adriamycin. Cytotoxicity of these agents has been shown to be potentiated by hyperbaric oxygen (Leifer , 2001; Monstrey et al,1997)

Adverse effects of HBO treatment include reversible myopia (Leach et al, 1998), barotrauma of the ear, claustrophobia (only in small treatment chambers), seizures (1.3 per 10 000 patient treatments), and, very rare, pulmonary oxygen toxicity (Bakker, 1984).Vasoconstiction, that could be expected due to the increased oxygen levels, was not observed in ischaemic or hypoxic tissues (Sheffield, 1988). Worsening of diabetic retinopathy could theoretically occur during hyperbaric oxygen therapy, but up until now this complication has not been reported.

2. Hyperbaric oxygen: mechanisms of action

The principle effect of hyperbaric oxygen treatment is creating hyperoxia in blood and tissues. Hyperbaric oxygen therapy implies administration of 100% under pressure greater than atmospheric. By raising the ambient pressure of oxygen either in the chamber or by breathing 100% oxygen through tight fitting mask, it is possible to increase the inspired PO_2 up to 3.0 bar. The most commonly used levels of inspired oxygen range from 2.4 to 2.8 bar. At these levels, amount of dissolved oxygen in plasma could potentially meet oxygen consumption requirements of the whole body. Hemoglobin remains saturated even in the venous capillary blood (Ramaswami &Lo, 2000). At 3 atmospheres of pressure, which is commonly used in the modern hyperbaric oxygen treatment, the alveolar oxygen pressure is about 2,180 mm Hg, the arterial oxygen tension is at least 1,800 mmHg, and tissue oxygen concentration is approximately 500 mmHg. High tissue oxygen concentration remains elevated for variable period of time (likely up to a few hours) after removal from hyperbaric chamber, which depends on tissue density and perfusion. (Sheridan & Shank,1999).

It has been demonstrated, that inhalation of O2 at pressures greater than 1 ATA will increase production of reactive oxygen species, which is fundamental for physiological mechanisms of numerous effects and also therapeutic mechanisms. (Thom,2009). Reactive oxygen species, as well as reactive nitrogen species, play important roles as signaling molecules in transduction cascades, or pathways for a variety of growth factors, cytokines, and hormonal substances.

3. Hyperbaric oxygen for chronic diabetic wound and ulcer healing

Diabetes mellitus is increasing in incidence and currently presents one of the major health problems worldwide. The total number of diabetic patients has been projected to increase from 171 million in 2000 to 366 million in 2030 (Wild et al, 2004), with concomitant rise of the major complications rate, among which chronic non-healing leg diabetic wounds, associated with vascular insufficiency du e to accelerated atherosclerotic process, is within area of this review focus. With this trend, the requirements for efficient treatment are obviously expected to increase exponentially.

The most prevalent forms of chronic wounds in diabetic patients are leg and foot ulcerations.(Leung, 2007; Tam & Moschella ,1991). Typical chronic, non-healing ischemic and diabetic wounds require prolonged time (more than 8 weeks) to heal, and sometimes do not heal or recur.

The pathophysiology of diabetic foot ulcer and its prolonged healing, however complex, has been extensively studied and is well described. Early development and accelerated progression of the lower extremity peripheral arterial atherosclerotic occlusive disease, with predilection to complete vascular blockade on the level distal to the knee, is a major causing factor. Other contributing factors include progressive development of sensory, vasomotor and autonomic neuropathy, alterations in autoregulation of dermal blood flow (Liu & Velazquez, 2008).It has been shown, that peripheral vascular disease (macroangiopathy), along with diabetic polyneuropathy, constitute the most important factors in the diabetic wound and ulcer development. About 20% of diabetic lower extremity ulcers have impaired arterial flow as primary ethiological factor, approximately 50 % associated with primary diabetic neuropathy, and up to 30% have both conditions (Reiber et al.,1999). Recently, microangiopathy has also been implicated in the pathogenesis of diabetic foot ulcers (La Fontaine et al.,2006; Ngo et al., 2005). Along with rapidly progressing atherosclerotic obstructive vascular disease, diabetic patients commonly exhibit an enhanced vascular responsiveness to vasoconstrictors, attenuated response to vasodilators and impaired regulation of blood flow in many different regions, from cerebral blood flow to local, dermal perfusion. Altered endothelial function of resistance vessels could contribute to altered regulation of regional blood flow and insufficient tissue perfusion in diabetes mellitus (Unfirer et al., 2008).

The fundamental role of oxygen in the physiology of wound healing is well documented (Brakora & Sheffield,1995; Hunt,1988). Measurement of the transcutaneous pressure of oxygen ($TcpO_2$) has been shown to be a valuable tool in predicting healing or non-healing in diabetic foot ulcers (Mathieu et al.,1990). It has been demonstrated, that patients with $TcpO_2$ values <20 mmHg, in comparison to patients with values >40 mmHg, have a 39-fold increase in failure of wound healing (Pecoraro, 1991, Bakker, 2000; Rollins et al., 2006). Hypoxia in the wound tissues promote the ulceration process, whereas a plentiful supply of oxygen is critically important for a variety of healing processes (Liu &Velazquez, 2008). Oxygen tension is positively correlated with key components of the healing process, such as angiogenesis (Knighton et al., 1983), collagen production (Hunt &Pai ,1972; Jonsson et al., 1991; Gurdol et al.,2010), bacterial elimination (Knighton et al., 1984;Cimsit et al.,2009) and epithelization (Uhl et al., 1994). In well-oxygenated wounds, all these components are greatly enhanced.

Of all other available oxygen delivery methods, hyperbaric oxygen therapy appears to be the most efficient option (Liu & Velazquez, 2008). Hyperbaric oxygen therapy has proved its efficiency in healing acceleration of ischemic and refractory diabetic wounds (Zamboni et al.,1997;Abidia et al., 2003; Hopf et al., 2005).

Despite the well-known beneficial effects of hyperbaric oxygen therapy on healing process of chronic ischemic and diabetic wounds and ulcers, its mechanisms of action are not completely understood. Restoring an adequate blood flow to the site of chronic wound is an essential prerequisite of successful healing response, which include modifying the altered vascular responsiveness to vasoactive substances and new vessel growth stimulation. It has been suggested, that hyperbaric oxygen is capable of induction of complex changes in the conducted vasomotor responses, thus modifying vascular sensitivity and reactivity to vasoactive substances (Drenjancević-Perić et al.,2009).It has also been hypothesized, that hyperbaric oxygen exerts beneficial effects on vascular function by affecting production or vessel sensitivity to vasoconstrictor and vasodilator metabolites of arachidonic acid and nitric oxide in response to physiological stimuli, namely acetylcholine, hypoxia and flow-mediated dilation, thus effectively restoring vascular reactivity (Unfirer et al., 2008). Available data is quite scarce and almost exclusively experimental. To date, no published results of large-scale, controlled prospective studies could be found.

Angiogenesis, in form of neovascularisation, is one of the essential processes that occur in the course of chronic diabetic wound healing. In conditions of hyperoxia, created by applying the hyperbaric oxygen therapy either locally (isolated extremity treatment) or generally in hyperbaric chamber, neovascularisation in hypoxic tissues occurs by two processes. Regional angiogenic stimuli increase the efficiency of new blood vessel growth by proliferation of microvascular endothelial cells, and also the recruitment and differentiation of circulation stem/progenitor cells (SPCs) to form vessels de novo. In clinically relevant concentrations, hyperbaric oxygen has been shown to influence both these processes (Thom, 2009). It has been demonstrated, that hyperbaric oxygen induces a cytoprotective and angiogenic response in human microvascular endothelial cells by increasing expression of immediate early and cytoprotective genes, which corresponded with increase in cell proliferation and oxidative stress resistance (Godman et al.,2010a,2010b).

Hyperbaric oxygen reduces circulating levels of proinflammatory cytokines, and also increases synthesis of many growth factors. Oxidative stress at the sites of neovascularization stimulates growth factors synthesis by augmenting synthesis and stabilizing hypoxia-inducible factor (HIF)-1. (Hunt et al.,2004, 2007) Vascular endothelial growth factor (VEGF) , angiopoetin and also stromal-derived factor-1 influence stromal cells differentiation to endothelial cells. VEGF, the most specific growth factor for neovascularization, has been shown to be increased by hyperbaric oxygen(Sheikh et all.,2000;Thom,2011).

Diabetic foot ulceration is a major predisposing factor for local infections, whereas various immunological disturbances and peripheral polyneuropathy play secondary roles. Diabetic foot ulcers are frequently polymicrobial with a high incidence of anaerobic organisms. Anaerobic infections are especially frequently seen in tissues with low oxygen tensions. Anaerobes are found in about 33% of cases of diabetic foot infections (Calhoun et al.,1992; Calhoun et al.,2002). Among the frequently isolated anaerobic organisms are species of *Bacteroides* and *Clostridia* (Boulton, 1988). Aerobic Gram-positive cocci (especially Staphylococcus aureus) are also among the most common, sometimes predominant, pathogens in diabetic foot infections. Patients with chronic wounds who are already receiving antibiotics, may be also infected with gram-positive rods, and those with established foot ischemia or gangrene may have obligate anaerobic pathogens (Lipsky et al., 2006).Hyperbaric oxygen therapy is often combined with antibiotics as an adjunctive treatment for various wound infections. Hyperoxia and hyperbaric oxygen exert antimicrobial effects by increasing the intracellular flux of reactive oxygen species. Hyperbaric oxygen may be either bacreiostatic or bactericidal for microorganisms that lack defenses against oxidants. In bacteria, reactive oxygen species cause DNA strand breaks, degradation of RNA, inhibition of amino acid biosynthesis, and inactivation of membrane transport proteins. Oxygen tensions also affect the activity of antimicrobial agents. In general, hyperoxia potentiates while anaerobiosis decreases the activity of many antimicrobial drugs. With regard to host defenses, hypoxia can seriously impair leukocyte bacterial killing function (Rabkin &Hunt ,1988; LaVan & Hunt ,1990). Hyperoxia elevates oxygen tensions in infected tissues to levels that facilitate oxygen-dependent killing by

leukocytes. Prolonged hyperoxia inhibits DNA synthesis in lymphocytes and impairs chemotactic activity, adherence, phagocytic capacity, and generation of the oxidative burst in polymorphonuclear leukocytes and macrophages. (Park et al., 1992; Cimsit, 2009).
One of the suggested criteria for hyperbaric oxygen therapy use is transcutaneous oxygen measurement of less than 40 mm Hg at the tissues surrounding the wound, most precisely, at the wound edges. This baseline measurement should be followed by testing the patient's tissue response to administration of 100% via tight face mask. The trascutaneous oxygen level should increase by at least 10 mm Hg to justify starting of hyperbaric oxygen therapy. After an hyperbaric oxygen trial, the transcutaneaous measurement should be greater than 200 mm Hg (Attinger, 2006; Hunter et al, 2010). It has been also demonstrated, that a transcutaneous oxygen tension (TcPO2) of 200 mmHg, measured in the peri-wound tissues while in-chamber, was the most effective determinant of success or failure of the therapy. It has been found , that TcPO2 in peri-wound tissues at sea level air of less than 15 mm Hg, together with a TcPO2 less than 400 mm Hg, measured in the same tissues in-chamber, proved to be most accurate predictor of hyperbaric oxygen therapy failure (reliability 75.8%, positive predictive value 73.3%)(Fife et all, 2002, 2007).
The commonly used protocols for hyperbaric oxygen therapy administration vary among institutions. No consensus has been reached so far in respect to single session and whole treatment duration. Most commonly, hyperbaric oxygen for diabetic wounds is administered at pressure range of 2 to 2.8 ATA, 5 days a week, with typical session duration of 45 to 90 minutes.(Wang, 2003). Other authors have been using daily treatments of 1.5 to 2 hours duration, for 20 to 40 days (Thom,2010).
The effectiveness of hyperbaric oxygen for diabetic and ischemic wounds treatment may be evaluated from prospective of two most important clinical outcomes: expediting the wound healing and reduction the amputation rate. Clinical efficacy of hyperbaric oxygen therapy in healing of chronic diabetic and ischemic wounds has been demonstrated by many researchers (Hinchliffe et al., 2008). Another group reported 90% healing in the intervention group *versus* 28% controls (Heng et all, 2000). The wound area reduction has been reported to occur at 2 weeks: 42% in the intervention group *versus* 21% (p = 0.037) and at 4 weeks: 62% *versus* 55% (Kessler et al., 2003). Two groups reported a favorable outcome after hyperbaric oxygen therapy in respect to expedited diabetic ulceration healing. One of groups has conducted a double-blind randomized trial, the main outcome of which was completely healed wound by 12 month after commencement of the therapy (2.5 ATA for 85 min, 5 days a week, for 8 weeks)in 52% of patients that received hyperbaric oxygen versus 29% of those from control group (Duzgun et al., 2008; Londahi et al.,2010,2011) .
It has been well demonstrated, that use of hyperbaric oxygen therapy was associated with decrease in amputation rate in diabetic patients. A decrease by 30% of major amputations rate in Wagner grade 4 patients has been reported in large prospective study (Faglia et al., 1996). Another study demonstrated even more significant (almost in 71%, 2 amputations in the study group versus 7 in control, a total of 30 patients) decrease of amputation rate (Doctor et al., 1992).

4. Hyperbaric oxygen in the treatment of necrotizing fasciitis and Fournier's gangrene

Necrotizing fasciitis has been defined as rapidly progressing life-threatening bacterial infection, that primarily involves skin and secondary subcutaneous tissues (Jallali et al.,

2005). Incidence of necrotizing fasciitis has increased over two decades (1980-2000), yet the disease still remains quite rare. The possible explanation may include increased microbial virulence and resistance because of excessive use of powerful antibiotics, and also possibly disease reporting and statistical work improvement (Sarani et al., 2009).

There are three basic subtypes of necrotizing fasciitis described. Approximately 55 to 75 % of type I caused by combination of gram-positive cocci, gram-negative rods, and anaerobes; less commonly, by species of bacteroides or Clostridium (Childers et al.,2002; Wong et al., 2003;Anaya &Dellinger, 2007). This type of infection tend to occur in the trunk and perineal areas and include Fournier's gangrene. Type II of necrotizing fasciitis mostly caused by monomicrobial flora, that include group A Streptococcus (S. pyogenes) alone or in association with Staphylococcus aureus. This type may be associated with toxic shock syndrome. During last 5 years, an increasing incidence of methicillin-resistant S. aureus (MRSA) is being reported, especially in IV drug users. Today, MRSA is cultured in approximately 40% of necrotic wounds (Miller et al., 2005; Maltezou & Giamarellou,2006;Thulin et al.,2006). Some sources classified necrotizing infection caused by Vibrio vulnificus as type III, although consensus regarding such classification remains yet to be reached. The biggest risk factors for this, the rarest, type of necrotizing fasciitis include exposure to warm sea water and also moderate to severe liver disease, particularly chronic hepatitis B (Howard et al., 1985).

Bacterial agents, that invade subcutaneous tissues through disrupted viscus of colorectal or urogenital area or perforated skin, rapidly spread over the adjacent tissues, producing endo- and exotoxins, that cause deep tissue ischemia and liquefactive necrosis that eventually lead to systemic disease (Salcido, 2007). Some of the exotoxins, namely M-1 and M-3 surface proteins, produced by S.aureus and Staphyloocci, increase microbial virulence by enhancing their ability to adhere to tissues and resistance to phagocytosis. Other exotoxins, namely A and B exert a variety of ill effects, that include endothelium damage, loss of microvascular integrity, increase of capillary permeability , causing plasma capillary leak, which results in tissue edema and impairment of capillary blood flow. These toxins, along with streptolysin O, stimulate CD4 cells and macrophages to produce large amounts of tumor necrosis factor-a,interleukin1 and 6 (Hackett & Stevens, 1992). Release of these cytokines into the circulation causes systemic inflammatory response and may lead to septic shock, multiorgan failure and eventual death. Superantigenes directly stimulate T-cells, causing activation of complement, bardykinin-kallikrein system and coagulation cascade, with small vessel thrombosis and tissue ischemia ensued (Salcido,2007).

Early radical surgical debridement along with aggressive, wide-spectrum antibiotic therapy remains a mainstay of the necrotizing fasciitis treatment. Despite the certain progress, achieved in this field, unfavorable outcome remains quite common.

High mortality rate of 20 to 40% (McHenry et al. ,1995) have prompted a search for effective ancillary methods of treatment to improve patients outcome. Hyperbaric oxygen therapy has shown some promising results, which promoted its use as an adjuvant therapeutic modality in this category of patients. Although variety of protocols have been employed, the most common method includes administration of oxygen at 2 to 3 ATA with average duration of 60 to 120 minutes. However, no consensus has been reached so far regarding either duration, timing or number of sessions, and established protocols for HBO therapy in necrotizing fasciitis or Fournier's gangrene are absent.

Most of clinical evidences, supporting the use of hyperbaric oxygen therapy, are of only anecdotal value at best. Most authors have chosen a decrease of the overall mortality rate as

an universal index of HBO therapy efficacy, reporting improved patients survival rates in majority of studies. The reported mortality rates varied significantly, from 0 to 33% (Jallali et al., 2005).
The lowest mortality rate ever reported, essentially zero deaths after combined early surgical debridement and HBO therapy in small group of only 9 patients with Fournier's gangrene, was shown in the early clinical study of (Eltorai et al.,1986). In this study, however, no data was provided either in respect to details of the treatment protocol details (duration of the study, number of sessions, time intervals between hyperbaric oxygen therapy sessions and surgical debridments). Another study included two series of 32 patients with clostridial gas gangrene and 11 patients wit perineal necrotizing fasciitis, who underwent hyperbaric oxygen therapy at 2.5 ATA for 120 minutes of session duration , and 3 first treatments were administered during first 24 hours after admission, and then repeated twice daily. The overall mortality rate was reported as 28% in gas gangrene group. In the group of patients treated with hyperbaric oxygen, 94% of the survivors healed completely and were able to walk normally (Him, 1993).
In yet another study, 33 patients were treated for perineal necrotizing fasciitis. Their management included wide early surgical debridment and drainage, massive antibiotic therapy and hyperbaric oxygen therapy at 2.5 ATA, 2 to12 times. The reported mortality rate was quite low (9.1%, 3 patients died out of 33) (Korhonen, 2000). Same group of researchers had also managed a group of 53 patients with Clostridial gas gangrene, and protocol here was pretty much identical to that used in patients with Fournier's gangrene. The reported mortality rate was 22.6%. In this study, substantially higher levels of subcutaneous PO2 at the same O2 pressures of 2.5 ATA during hyperbaric oxygen therapy were found in the vicinity of infected areas than in healthy tissues. Authors concluded, that hyperbaric oxygen therapy appears to be life-, limb, and tissue saving, and that the hyperoxygenation of tissue zone surrounding the infected area may be of significance in preventing the expansion of microorganisms. (Korhonen at al., 1999, 2000). Authors of another study administered hyperbaric oxygen shortly (about 7 hours) after surgical debridement, which resulted in achievement of only 12.5% mortality rate. However, no control group was mentioned in this study, which makes it difficult to draw a definite conclusion regarding the net effect of the hyperbaric oxygen therapy (Gozal et al., 1986) In the controlled study, included group of 17 patients that received hyperbaric oxygen along with surgical debridement and antibiotics versus that of 12 patients, whose treatment did not include hyperbaric oxygen therapy, use of this modality has allowed to decrease overall mortality from 66% to 23%. This result has been achieved despite the fact, that patients received hyperbaric oxygen, were more seriously ill (some of them were in septic shock), which makes the beneficial effect of the therapy in this study particularly noteworthy (Riseman et al., 1990). In larger, albeit without control group study, efficacy of including HBOT in the treatment protocol in 42 consecutive patients has been proved by decreasing of overall mortality from 34%(national reported rate) to 11.9%, with 0% amputations (vs.50% of national average) in hyperbaric oxygen-treated patients (Escobar et all, 2005)
A growing number of studies, in contrast with those reported positive results of hyperbaric oxygen therapy, have demonstrated lack of any advantages of the hyperbaric oxygen therapy. In the large controlled multicenter study, (Brown et al.,1994), hyperbaric oxygen therapy was not associated with statistically significant decrease in mortality (30% in HBO group vs. 42% in control), number of debridements (2.4 in hyperbaric oxygen

group vs 1.3 in control) was actually higher, and length of hospital stay was not different between groups(31.6 days in hyperbaric oxygen vs. 31.3 days in control). In this study, however, majority of the patients (66%) received less than 4 sessions, which potentially makes the impact of hyperbaric oxygen therapy substantially weaker. Also, patients who were selected for hyperbaric oxygen therapy, had more advanced stages of sepsis, which potentially may have introduce a bias factor in the results interpretation. Authors of another study found no differences in length of hospital stay, complications rate and mortality between groups of patients with necrotizing fasciitis, where one was treated with hyperbaric oxygen therapy, and another wasn't; however, 25% of non- hyperbaric oxygen therapy group required amputations, whereas patients from hyperbaric oxygen therapy group needed no such intervention (Hassan et al.,2010). Authors of the retrospective study, reviewing 10-year - long experience of using HBOT as an adjuvant treatment for necrotizing fasciitis, found no improvements from hyperbaric oxygen use, but rather worsening of results in respect to mortality rate (36% in hyperbaric oxygen therapy group vs. 25% in control), number of debridements (2.5 with hyperbaric oxygen therapy vs 1.5 in controls). Difference in length of hospital stay, which was, however, shorter in hyperbaric oxygen therapy group (15.9 vs 20 days in controls), was not statistically significant.

Another retrospective study revealed considerably higher mortality among the patients with Fournier's gangrene, treated with hyperbaric oxygen therapy, in comparison with those received no such treatment (26.9 vs 12.5%). The potential reason for this finding, again, may be attributed to the selection of the much sicker patients for hyperbaric oxygen therapy (Mindrup et al., 2005).

Absolute majority, if not all, of studies investigating the effects of hyperbaric oxygen therapy, are retrospective ones. Even the largest series include several dozen patients at best, with most common sample size around 20 patients, either in study or control groups. Such small numbers of subjects preclude the use of vigorous statistical methods in comparison studies, investigating mortality and morbidity rates, tissue- and limb- salvage efficacy of the hyperbaric oxygen therapy. These limitations substantially diminish the predictive value of quite scarce published studies.

To date, even after thorough literature research, we could not find any prospective, randomized comparison study investigating different effects of hyperbaric oxygen therapy. Regretfully, it appears that truly robust proof of either positive or negative effect of hyperbaric oxygen therapy, at least as an adjuvant therapy for necrotizing fasciitis and gangrene, is currently absent.

There are numerous reasons to this situation. Scarcity of the resources (many hospitals do not possess the hyperbaric oxygenation chambers), lack of established guidelines, differences on clinical protocols (outlining timing, number of sessions, time correlation with debridements , and more), clinicians' opinions and experience, and also tendency to reserve the hyperbaric oxygen therapy, a quite expensive method, for the sickest, critically ill, oftentimes frankly moribund patients, are among the important limiting factors, making it truly difficult to elucidate the genuine impact of hyperbaric oxygen therapy in practically every area of its use (Jallali et al., 2005). In its current status, based on existent level of pro— and contra- evidences, HBOT efficacy remains controversial at best, and may not be unanimously recommended as therapeutic modality in every case of necrotizing fasciitis or gangrene.

5. Conclusion

Diabetic foot chronic wounds and ulcerations adjuvant treatment with hyperbaric oxygen appears to be efficient with respect to promoted healing and also in decrease of major amputations rate.

Hyperbaric oxygen therapy may not replace the combination of early aggressive debridements and wide-spectrum antibiotic therapy, but rather remains an adjuvant, however sometimes efficient, method in the management of necrotizing fasciitis and gangrene.

6. References

Abidia A, Laden G, Kuhan G, Johnson BF, Wilkinson AR, Renwick PM, Masson EA &McCollum PT. (2003)The role of hyperbaric oxygen therapy in ischaemic diabetic lower extremity ulcers: a double-blind randomised-controlled trial. *Eur J Vasc Endovasc Surg*.25,6,((Jun 2003),pp.513-8

Anaya DA, Dellinger EP.(2007) Necrotizing soft-tissue infection: diagnosis and management. *Clin Infect Dis.* 44,5,(Mar 2007),pp.705-10

Attinger CE, Janis JE, Steinberg J, Schwartz J, Al-Attar A & Couch K.(2006) Clinical approach to wounds: débridement and wound bed preparation including the use of dressings and wound-healing adjuvants. *Plast Reconstr Surg.* 117, 7 Suppl, (Jan 2006),pp.72S-109S

Bakker DJ(1984). The use of hyperbaric oxygen in the treatment of certain infectious diseases especially gas gangrene and acute dermal gangrene (Dissertation). *University of Amsterdam: Wageningen, The Netherlands,* 1984.

Bakker DJ (2000)Hyperbaric oxygen therapy and the diabetic foot. *Diabetes Metab Res Rev.* 16 Suppl 1 (Sep-Oct 2000),pp.S55-8

Boulton AJ.(1988) The diabetic foot. *Med Clin North Am 72,6,(Nov 1988),pp.1513-30*

Brakora MJ, Sheffield PJ (1995). Hyperbaric oxygen therapy for diabetic wounds. *Clin Podiatr Med Surg* 12, (1995)*pp.* 105–117.

Brown DR, Davis NL, Lepawsky M, Cunningham J & Kortbeek J.(1994) A multicenter review of the treatment of major truncal necrotizing infections with and without hyperbaric oxygen therapy. *Am J Surg*.167,5,(May 1994),pp.485-9

Calhoun JH, Mader JT & Sanford JP. (1992)Infection in the diabetic foot. *Hosp Pract (Off Ed)* 27,3A,(Mar 1992),pp.81-4,87-90,99 passim

Calhoun JH, Overgaard KA, Stevens CM, Dowling JP & Mader JT.(2009) Diabetic foot ulcers and infections: current concepts. *Adv Skin Wound Care.* 15,1,(Jan-Feb 2002),pp.31-42

Childers BJ, Potyondy LD, Nachreiner R, Rogers FR, Childers ER, Oberg KC, Hendricks DL &Hardesty RA.(2003) Necrotizing fasciitis: a fourteen-year retrospective study of 163 consecutive patients. *J Bone Joint Surg Am.* 85-A,8,(Aug 2003),pp.1454-60

Cimşit M, Uzun G & Yildiz S.(2009) Hyperbaric oxygen therapy as an anti-infective agent. *Expert Rev Anti Infect Ther7,8,(Oct 2009),pp.1015-26*

Doctor N, Pandya S& Supe A.(1992) Hyperbaric oxygen therapy in diabetic foot. *J Postgrad Med.* 38,3,(Jul-Sep 1992),pp.112-4

Drenjancević-Perić I, Gros M & Kibel A.(2009) Influence of hyperbaric oxygen on blood vessel reactivity: concept of changes in conducted vasomotor response. *Coll Antropol 33,2,(Jun 2009),pp.681-5*

Duzgun AP, Satir HZ, Ozozan O, Saylam B, Kulah B &Coskun F.(2008) Effect of hyperbaric oxygen therapy on healing of diabetic foot ulcers. *J Foot Ankle Surg.* 47,6, (Nov-Dec 2008),pp.515-9

Eltorai IM, Hart GB, Strauss MB, Montroy R & Juler GL.(1986) The role of hyperbaric oxygen in the management of Fournier's gangrene. *Int Surg.* 71,1,(Jan-Mar 1986),pp.53-8

Escobar SJ, Slade JB Jr, Hunt TK, Cianci P. Adjuvant hyperbaric oxygen therapy (HBO2)for treatment of necrotizing fasciitis reduces mortality and amputation rate. *Undersea Hyperb Med.* 32,6,(Nov-Dec 2005), pp.437-43

Faglia E, Favales F, Aldeghi A, Calia P, Quarantiello A, Oriani G, Michael M, Campagnoli P & Morabito A.(1996) Adjunctive systemic hyperbaric oxygen therapy in treatment of severe prevalently ischemic diabetic foot ulcer. A randomized study. *Diabetes Care.* 19,12,(Dec 1996),pp.1338-43

Fife CE, Buyukcakir C, Otto GH, Sheffield PJ, Warriner RA, Love TL & Mader J.(2002) The predictive value of transcutaneous oxygen tension measurement in diabetic lower extremity ulcers treated with hyperbaric oxygen therapy: a retrospective analysis of 1,144 patients. *Wound Repair Regen.* 10,4,(Jul-Aug 2002),pp.198-207

Fife CE, Buyukcakir C, Otto G, Sheffield P, Love T &Warriner R 3rd.(2007) Factors influencing the outcome of lower-extremity diabetic ulcers treated with hyperbaric oxygen therapy. *Wound Repair Regen.* 15,3,(May-Jun 2007),pp.322-31

Foster JH.(1992) Hyperbaric oxygen therapy: contraindications and complications. *J Oral Maxillofac Surg.*50 ,10,(Oct.1992),pp.1081-66

Godman CA, Joshi R, Giardina C, Perdrizet G &Hightower LE.(2009) Hyperbaric oxygen treatment induces antioxidant gene expression. *Ann N Y Acad Sci.*1197,(Jun 2009),pp.178-83

Godman CA, Chheda KP, Hightower LE, Perdrizet G, Shin DG &Giardina C.(2010) Hyperbaric oxygen induces a cytoprotective and angiogenic response in human microvascular endothelial cells. *Cell Stress Chaperones.* 15,4,(Jul 2010),pp.431-42

Gozal D, Ziser A, Shupak A, Ariel A & Melamed Y.(1986) Necrotizing fasciitis. *Arch Surg.* 121,2,(Feb 1986),pp.233-5

Gurdol F, Cimsit M, Oner-Iyidogan Y, Kocak H, Sengun S&Yalcinkaya-Demirsoz S.(2010) Collagen synthesis, nitric oxide and asymmetric dimethylarginine in diabetic subjects undergoing hyperbaric oxygen therapy. *Physiol Res 59,3,(Aug 2010),pp.423-9*

Hackett SP, Stevens DL. Streptococcal toxic shock syndrome: synthesis of tumor necrosis factor and interleukin-1 by monocytes stimulated with pyrogenic exotoxin A and streptolysin O. *J Infect Dis.* 165,5,(May 1992),pp.879-85

Hassan Z, Mullins RF, Friedman BC, Shaver JR, Brandigi C, Alam B & Mian MA.(2010) Treating necrotizing fasciitis with or without hyperbaric oxygen therapy. *Undersea Hyperb Med.* 37,2,(Mar-Apr 2010),pp.115-23

Heng MC, Harker J, Csathy G, Marshall C, Brazier J, Sumampong S & Paterno Gomez E.(2000) Angiogenesis in necrotic ulcers treated with hyperbaric oxygen. *Ostomy Wound Manage.* 46,9,(Sep 2000),p.18-28,30-2

Him M.(1993) Hyperbaric oxygen in the treatment of gas gangrene and perineal necrotizing fasciitis. A clinical and experimental study. *Eur J Surg Suppl.* 570,(1993),pp.1-36

Hinchliffe RJ, Valk GD, Apelqvist J, Armstrong DG, Bakker K, Game FL, Hartemann-Heurtier A, Löndahl M, Price PE, van Houtum WH &Jeffcoate WJ.(2008) A systematic review of the effectiveness of interventions to enhance the healing of chronic ulcers of the foot in diabetes. *Diabetes Metab Res Rev 24 Suppl 1,(May-Jun 2008), pp.S119-44*

Hopf HW, Gibson JJ, Angeles AP, Constant JS, Feng JJ, Rollins MD, Zamirul Hussain M& Hunt TK. Hyperoxia and angiogenesis. *Wound Repair Regen 13,6,(Nov-Dec 2005),pp.558-64*

Howard RJ, Pessa ME, Brennaman BH & Ramphal R.(1985) Necrotizing soft-tissue infections caused by marine vibrios. *Surgery.* 98,1,(Jul 1985),pp.126-30

Hunt TK, Pai MP.(1972) The effect of varying ambient oxygen tensions on wound metabolism and collagen synthesis. *Surg Gynecol Obstet.* 135,4,(Oct 1972),pp.561-7

Hunt TK, Ellison EC & Sen CK.(2004) Oxygen: at the foundation of wound healing--introduction. *World J Surg.*28,3,(Mar 2004),pp.291-3

Hunt TK, Aslam RS, Beckert S, Wagner S, Ghani QP, Hussain MZ, Roy S & Sen CK.(2007) Aerobically derived lactate stimulates revascularization and tissue repair via redox mechanisms. *Antioxid Redox Signal.*9,8,(Aug 2007),pp.1115-24

Hunt TK (2008) The physiology of wound healing. *Med Hypotheses 71,7, (Nov.2008),pp.776-80*

Hunter S, Langemo DK, Anderson J, Hanson D &Thompson P.(2010) Hyperbaric oxygen therapy for chronic wounds. *Adv Skin Wound Care.*23,3,(Mar 2010),p.116-9

Jallali N, Withey S & Butler PE.(2005) Hyperbaric oxygen as adjuvant therapy in the management of necrotizing fasciitis. *Am J Surg.* 189,4,(Apr 2005),pp.462-6

Jonsson K, Jensen JA, Goodson WH 3rd, Scheuenstuhl H, West J, Hopf HW& Hunt TK.(1991) Tissue oxygenation, anemia, and perfusion in relation to wound healing in surgical patients. *Ann Surg 214,5, (Nov 1991),pp.605-13*

Kessler L, Bilbault P, Ortéga F, Grasso C, Passemard R, Stephan D, Pinget M & Schneider F.(2003) Hyperbaric oxygenation accelerates the healing rate of nonischemic chronic diabetic foot ulcers: a prospective randomized study. *Diabetes Care.* 26,8,(Aug 2003),pp.2378-82

Knighton DR, Hunt TK, Scheuenstuhl H, Halliday BJ, Werb Z & Banda MJ(1983). Oxygen tension regulates the expression of angiogenesis factor by macrophages. *Science.*221,4617, (Sep 1983),pp.1283-5

Knighton DR, Halliday B & Hunt TK. Oxygen as an antibiotic. The effect of inspired oxygen on infection. *Arch Surg119,2,(Feb 1984),pp.199-204*

Korhonen K, Kuttila K & Niinikoski J.(1999) Subcutaneous tissue oxygen and carbon dioxide tensions during hyperbaric oxygenation: an experimental study in rats. *Eur J Surg.* 165,9,(Sep 1999),pp.885-90

Korhonen K.(2000) Hyperbaric oxygen therapy in acute necrotizing infections. With a special reference to the effects on tissue gas tensions. *Ann Chir Gynaecol.* 89 Suppl 214, (Mar 2000),pp.7-36

Korhonen K, Kuttila K &Niinikoski J.(2000) Tissue gas tensions in patients with necrotising fasciitis and healthy controls during treatment with hyperbaric oxygen: a clinical study. *Eur J Surg.* 166,7,(Jul 2000),pp.530-4

La Fontaine J, Harkless LB, Davis CE, Allen MA & Shireman PK.(1999) Current concepts in diabetic microvascular dysfunction. *Diabetes Care*.22,1,(Jan 1999),pp.157-62

LaVan FB, Hunt TK. Oxygen and wound healing. *Clin Plast Surg*. 17,3,(Jul 1990),pp.453-72

Leifer G (2001)Hyperbaric oxygen therapy. *Am J Nurs*. 101, 8, (Aug 2001),pp.26-34

Leach RM, Rees PJ & Wilmshurst P.(1998) Hyperbaric oxygen therapy. *BMJ* 317,(Oct 24 1998)pp-no data

Leung PC. (2004)Diabetic foot ulcers--a comprehensive review. *Diabetes Care*.27,5,(May 2004),pp.1047-53

Lipsky BA, Berendt AR, Deery HG, Embil JM, Joseph WS, Karchmer AW, LeFrock JL, Lew DP, Mader JT, Norden C, Tan JS; Infectious Diseases Society of America. Diagnosis and treatment of diabetic foot infections. *Plast Reconstr Surg*.117,7Suppl,(Jun 2006), pp.212S-238S

Liu ZJ, Velazquez OC.(1991) Hyperoxia, endothelial progenitor cell mobilization, and diabetic wound healing. *Cardiol Clin*.9,3,(Aug1991),pp.555-63

Löndahl M, Katzman P, Nilsson A & Hammarlund C.(2010)Hyperbaric oxygen therapy facilitates healing of chronic foot ulcers in patients with diabetes. *Diabetes Care*. 33,5,(May 2010),pp.998-1003

Löndahl M, Katzman P, Hammarlund C, Nilsson A & Landin-Olsson M.(2011) Relationship between ulcer healing after hyperbaric oxygen therapy and transcutaneous oximetry, toe blood pressure and ankle-brachial index in patients with diabetes and chronic foot ulcers. *Diabetologia*. 65,8,(Jan 2011),pp.65-8

Maltezou HC, Giamarellou H.(2006) Community-acquired methicillin-resistant Staphylococcus aureus infections. *Int J Antimicrob Agents*. 27,2,(Feb 2006),pp.87-96

Mathieu D, Wattel F, Bouachour G, Billard V&Defoin JF.(1990) Post-traumatic limb ischemia: prediction of final outcome by transcutaneous oxygen measurements in hyperbaric oxygen. *J Trauma*.30,3,(Mar 1990),pp.307-14

McHenry CR, Piotrowski JJ, Petrinic D& Malangoni MA.(1995) Determinants of mortality for necrotizing soft-tissue infections. *Ann Surg*. 221,5,(May 1995),pp.558-63, discussion 563-5

Miller LG, Perdreau-Remington F, Rieg G, Mehdi S, Perlroth J, Bayer AS, Tang AW, Phung TO & Spellberg B.(2005)Necrotizing fasciitis caused by community-associated methicillin-resistant Staphylococcus aureus in Los Angeles. *N Engl J Med*. 352,14,(Apr 7 2005),pp.1445-53

Mindrup SR, Kealey GP & Fallon B.(2005) Hyperbaric oxygen for the treatment of fournier's gangrene. *J Urol*. 173,6,(Jun 2005),pp.1975-7

Monstrey SJ, Mullick P, Narayanan K & Ramasastry SS. (1997)Hyperbaric oxygen therapy and free radical production: an experimental study in doxorubicin (Adriamycin) extravasation injuries. *Ann Plast Surg*.38,2,(Feb.1997),pp.163-8

Ngo BT, Hayes KD, DiMiao DJ, Srinivasan SK, Huerter CJ & Rendell MS.(2005) Manifestations of cutaneous diabetic microangiopathy. *Am J Clin Dermatol*. 6,4,(2005),pp.225-37

Park MK, Myers RA & Marzella L.(1992)Oxygen tensions and infections: modulation of microbial growth, activity of antimicrobial agents, and immunologic responses. *Clin Infect Dis*. 14,3,(Mar 1992),pp.720-40

Pecoraro RE.(1991) The nonhealing diabetic ulcer--a major cause for limb loss. *Prog Clin Biol Res.* 365,(1991),pp.27-43

Rabkin JM, Hunt TK. (1987)Local heat increases blood flow and oxygen tension in wounds. *Arch Surg.* 122,2,(Feb 1987),pp.221-5

Ramaswami RA, Lo WK.(2000)Use of hyperbaric oxygen therapy in Hong Kong *HKMJ,* 6,1,(2000)pp.108-112

Reiber GE, Vileikyte L, Boyko EJ, del Aguila M, Smith DG, Lavery LA & Boulton AJ.(2006) Causal pathways for incident lower-extremity ulcers in patients with diabetes from two settings. *J Am Podiatr Med Assoc.* 96,3,(May-Jun 2006),pp.245-52

Riseman JA, Zamboni WA, Curtis A, Graham DR, Konrad HR & Ross DS.(1990) Hyperbaric oxygen therapy for necrotizing fasciitis reduces mortality and the need for debridements. *Surgery.* 108,5,(Nov 1990),pp.847-50

Rollins MD, Gibson JJ, Hunt TK &Hopf HW.(2006) Wound oxygen levels during hyperbaric oxygen treatment in healing wounds. *Undersea Hyperb Med.* 33,1,(Jan-Feb 2006),pp.17-25

Salcido RS. Necrotizing fasciitis: reviewing the causes and treatment strategies. *Adv Skin Wound Care.* 20,5,(May 2007),pp.288-93

Sarani B, Strong M, Pascual J & Schwab CW.(2002) Necrotizing fasciitis: current concepts and review of the literature. *Am Surg.*68,2,(Feb 2002),pp.109-16

Sheikh AY, Gibson JJ, Rollins MD, Hopf HW, Hussain Z & Hunt TK.(2000) Effect of hyperoxia on vascular endothelial growth factor levels in a wound model. *Arch Surg.* 135,11,(Nov 2000),pp.1293-7

Sheffield PJ. *(1988)*Tissue oxygen measurements. *In: Problem Wounds: The Role of Oxygen, (*Davis JC, Hunt TK*). pp.*17–51,*Elsevier: (ISBN-no data)* New York and Amsterdam.

Sheridan RL, Shank ES.(1999) Hyperbaric oxygen treatment: a brief overview of a controversial topic. *The Journal of Trauma: Injury, Infection and Critical care* 47,2,(Aug 1999) pp.426-435

Tam M, Moschella SL.(1991) Vascular skin ulcers of limbs. *Cardiol Clin.* 9,3,(Aug 1991),pp.555-63

Thom SR.(2009) Oxidative stress is fundamental to hyperbaric oxygen therapy. *J Appl Physiol.* 106,3,(Mar 2009),pp.988-95

Thom SR.(2011) Hyperbaric oxygen: its mechanisms and efficacy. *Plast Reconstr Surg* 127 Suppl 1,(Jan 2011),pp.131S-141S

Thulin P, Johansson L, Low DE, Gan BS, Kotb M, McGeer A & Norrby-Teglund A.(2006) Viable group A streptococci in macrophages during acute soft tissue infection. *PLoS Med.* 3,3,(Mar 2006),e53

Uhl E, Sirsjö A, Haapaniemi T, Nilsson G & Nylander G.(1994) Hyperbaric oxygen improves wound healing in normal and ischemic skin tissue. *Plast Reconstr Surg.* 93,4,(Apr 1994),pp.835-41

Unfirer S, Kibel A& Drenjancevic-Peric I.(2008) The effect of hyperbaric oxygen therapy on blood vessel function in diabetes mellitus. *Med Hypotheses.* 71,5,(Nov 2008), pp.776-80.

Wang C, Schwaitzberg S, Berliner E, Zarin DA& Lau J.(2003) Hyperbaric oxygen for treating wounds: a systematic review of the literature. *Arch Surg.* 138,3,(Mar 2003),pp.272-9

Wild S, Roglic G, Green A, Sicree R& King H.(2007) Global prevalence of diabetes: estimates for the year 2000 and projections for 2030. *Surgeon*.5,4,(Aug 2007)pp.219-31

Wong CH, Chang HC, Pasupathy S, Khin LW, Tan JL& Low CO.(2009) Necrotizing fasciitis: clinical presentation, microbiology, and determinants of mortality. *J Am Coll Surg*. 208,2,(Feb 2009),pp.279-88

Zamboni WA, Wong HP, Stephenson LL& Pfeifer MA.(1997) Evaluation of hyperbaric oxygen for diabetic wounds: a prospective study. *Undersea Hyperb Med*.24,3,(Sep 1997),pp.175-9